"I love this book! Tasha has outdone herself with this easy-to-understand, level-headed, and straightforward guide to doing keto as a woman. A much-needed resource, tailored specifically to women's physiology and healthy endocrine function, it is full of insight into how to use keto to optimize our metabolic rate training, build strength, and enhance body composition. I would highly recommend this book to any women seeking to master keto and learn valuable tools and insights along the way!"

—**Vanessa Spina**, author of *Keto Essentials*

"*Keto: A Woman's Guide*, is a must-read for all women wanting to win the weight loss battle with a keto lifestyle! Regular hormonal changes make the female approach to weight loss different than a standard keto plan geared towards men. This guide helps women understand why their male counterparts seem to struggle less when it comes to losing weight. Tasha does an excellent job explaining how things like hunger and metabolic rate can fluctuate during the female hormonal cycle. "

—**Lisa MarcAurele**, founder of Low Carb Yum

"A keto book for women, by a woman; this is just what the keto community needed. We've known for decades that women's bodies have different metabolic pathways for various drugs and medicines, why would it be any different for the food we eat? *Keto: A Woman's Guide* helps identify the benefits and potential pitfalls of the female keto lifestyle and set women up for greater success."

—**Carolyn Ketchum**, best-selling author of *The Everyday Ketogenic Kitchen*

"Tasha's book should be on every keto woman's bookshelf. Men and women are so different when it comes to losing weight, yet most advice on how to follow a healthy diet is not designed for their respective needs. From understanding how female hormones impact weight loss and ketosis to the smartest food and exercise strategies, Tasha explains everything in such simple terms you'll be able to start your low-carb journey right away."

—**Martina Slajerova**, bestselling author of *The Beginner's KetoDiet Cookbook*

"Whether we realize it or not, keto is different for men and women. With her nutrition expertise and her extensive experience with the keto diet, I can't think of a better person than Tasha to write this much-needed book. I highly recommend *Keto: A Woman's Guide* to any woman serious about understanding her body and following keto the right way."

—**Maya Krampf**, founder Wholesome Yum

"*Keto: A Women's Guide* is going to be my new resource for women wanting to adopt the ketogenic diet. As a low-carb athlete, I appreciate that exercise and athletic training is covered in this invaluable guide, as this topic alone can be quite tricky to navigate as you venture from the world of high carb sports nutrition into the wonderful realm of keto."

—**Aaron Day**, creator of FatForWeight Loss

"Tasha provides a voice of reason in a world of keto confusion. She expertly counters myths around the ketogenic diet and set her readers up for long-term success. "

—**Annissa Slusher**, creator of Simply So Healthy

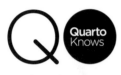

Inspiring | Educating | Creating | Entertaining

Brimming with creative inspiration, how-to projects, and useful information to enrich your everyday life, Quarto Knows is a favorite destination for those pursuing their interests and passions. Visit our site and dig deeper with our books into your area of interest: Quarto Creates, Quarto Cooks, Quarto Homes, Quarto Lives, Quarto Drives, Quarto Explores, Quarto Gifts, or Quarto Kids.

First Published in 2020 by Fair Winds Press, an imprint of The Quarto Group,
100 Cummings Center, Suite 265-D, Beverly, MA 01915, USA.
T (978) 282-9590 F (978) 283-2742 QuartoKnows.com

Fair Winds Press titles are also available at discount for retail, wholesale, promotional, and bulk purchase. For details, contact the Special Sales Manager by email at specialsales@quarto.com or by mail at The Quarto Group, Attn: Special Sales Manager, 100 Cummings Center, Suite 265-D, Beverly, MA 01915, USA.

24 23 22 21 20   1 2 3 4 5

ISBN: 978-1-59233-888-7

Digital edition published in 2020
eISBN: 978-1-63159-752-7

Library of Congress Cataloging-in-Publication Data is available.

Cover, page design, and illustrations: Tanja Jacobson, crsld.co
Photography: Tasha Metcalf

Printed in China

The information in this book is for educational purposes only. It is not intended to replace the advice of a physician or medical practitioner. Please see your health-care provider before beginning any new health program.

Creator of Ketogasm

TASHA METCALF

KETO

A Woman's Guide & Cookbook

The Groundbreaking Program For
Effective Fat-Burning, Weight Loss
& Hormonal Balance

FAIR WINDS

CONTENTS

IMPLEMENTATION OF THE KETO DIET 107

RECIPES 187

Introduction

This book is the first of its kind: a nutritional guidebook for keto explicitly written with the female body in mind. Women are biologically different from men—from our body composition to our cyclical hormonal fluctuations and right down to our chromosomes. The way our bodies burn fuel is dissimilar: Our metabolism seesaws from week to week, and our eating behavior is primarily driven by hormones that urge us to indulge beyond our needs on a regular basis.

We face different challenges than men, so why follow the same dieting advice? This book aims to bridge the gap between keto diet "rules" and what women restricting carbohydrates need—setting realistic expectations, variations, and actionable strategies along the way. This book will teach you how to develop increased metabolic flexibility using the keto diet and how to tailor your way of eating for optimal fat loss, hormonal balance, and long-term success.

In other words, you will learn to make keto work for *you*.

Part one of this book teaches you about the keto diet and fat-burning metabolism, while myth busting common misconceptions and addressing diet dogma. This sets the stage for you to confidently approach your diet, avoid the pitfalls, and put the naysayers to rest.

In part two, you will learn how female energy dynamics and hormones can make or break your effort to lose weight. You will learn how the keto diet and calories coexist, how the menstrual cycle and menopause affect metabolism and eating behavior, and how the keto diet can be used to bring harmony to your hormones.

The final part of the book focuses on implementation, bringing everything you have learned in the previous chapters to life with easy-to-follow strategies and instructions. You will discover a clear plan of action to improve your body composition and heal hormonal imbalances one step at a time.

—

After using keto to manage my weight and heal my body, I am grateful for the opportunity to present here a detailed plan to help you do the same. Although this book is intended for you to learn and take action, it is also a reflection on the things I would have done differently when transitioning from a high-carb diet. Consider this book a culmination of everything I wish I had known when starting keto years ago.

If you are ready to take charge of your health and transform your body, this friendly guide will help you along your journey. If you feel overwhelmed, know you are stronger and far more capable than you realize. Keto has profoundly transformed my life, and I hope it can do the same for you. If I can do it, I know you can, too. Now let's get started.

KETO IN CONTEXT

Laying the groundwork for what is to come, part one walks you through the fundamentals of what keto is—and is not.

In chapter 1 you will learn where keto fits compared to other low-carb diets and the various ways to achieve nutritional ketosis. You may be surprised to learn there is more than one approach to the keto diet, and the one most buzzed about in the media may not actually apply to you!

Diving straight into macronutrients, or "macros," chapter 2 will help you understand where our energy comes from and how its sources affect our overall health, metabolism, and body composition. You will quickly learn not all calories are created equal.

If you still have doubts about choosing a fat-fueled diet, chapter 3 will put your fears to rest. You will learn why carbs and fats don't mix, how to become an effective fat-burner, and what benefits accompany the new metabolic adaptations of burning fat. To make sure you start off on the right foot, we'll also tackle the biggest keto myths surrounding this way of eating—they aren't what you think!

1

What Is Keto?

Keto is a truncated version of the word **keto**genic, which refers to a diet that relies on the metabolic state of nutritional **keto**sis, in which your body runs off fat and **keto**nes instead of sugar. It's just a cute little nickname—get it? Don't worry; we'll get into what all that other stuff means, too.

A ketogenic diet significantly reduces carbohydrate intake and replaces the lost source of energy with fat. This reduction in carbs puts your body into a metabolic state called *ketosis*. Just so we're all on the same page, the important takeaway here is that carbohydrate restriction is what induces ketosis, not fat consumption.

Once the body is in ketosis, it becomes increasingly proficient at burning fat for energy. It also turns fat into ketones in the liver, which provides another form of energy for the body. The fat our body is using for fuel can come from the foods we eat, but it can also come from fat stored in adipose tissue when our diet doesn't meet our daily caloric needs.[1] Adipose tissue is your body fat—your muffin top, love handles, and double chin are literally stored energy waiting to be burned when your body needs it.

With continued carbohydrate restriction and long-term ketosis, cells in the body ultimately shift to preferentially using more fat and ketones in place of sugar. We will dive further into the science behind these adaptations in upcoming chapters, but this is the basic idea behind a standard keto diet.

The typical description of a ketogenic diet revolves around the concept of low carb, high fat, and moderate protein. Without any context, these terms are relative at best. How little is "low"? Does "high" mean the sky's the limit? Where does "moderate" stack up against what you typically eat? These seemingly straightforward questions are deceptively tricky to answer. It's nearly impossible to offer a precise quantitative definition because there is currently no consensus.

The lack of consensus is the result of boundless variables that alter recommendations on a case-by-case basis. That goes double for women, as our physiology tends to complicate things even further. My point isn't that we are too complex to figure out what to eat—just that we're all unique and there is no one-size-fits-all approach to nutrition and dieting.

This book is intended for women using nutritional ketosis as a dieting strategy to balance hormones and improve body composition. But keeping in mind that everyone is different, we'll cover possible modifications to the standard ketogenic diet so you can shape a plan that works for you—not your friend who told you about keto, not the girl with the giant social media following, not the guy at the gym, not me, Y-O-U.

We'll use the following interpretation of low carb, high fat, and moderate protein as a general framework:

Low Carb: Carbohydrates are restricted to achieve nutritional ketosis.

High Fat: Most energy needs are met with fat. If your goal is to reduce body fat, both dietary fat and adipose tissue will satisfy caloric needs.

Moderate Protein: Protein intake adequately meets the body's requirements.

The Vast World of Low-Carb Diets

Now let's explore how we have arrived at the modern-day keto craze. By looking at some historical and present-day diets focused on carbohydrate restriction, we can gain a broader understanding of where keto fits in.

Ancestral Diets and Available Fuel Sources

To gain historical perspective, we need to look at hunting and fishing cultures of indigenous peoples. Before the explosion of agriculture, people hunted for their food. Our ancestors were opportunistic eaters, meaning they ate what was available to them. They hunted, fished, and gathered whatever they could, whenever they could, wherever they could. If they had meat and fish available, that's what they consumed. If they were able to find fruit, they ate that as well. Humans as a species have evolved to switch between fuel sources based on food availability, which is a fundamental survival mechanism.

My point isn't that we are too complex to figure out what to eat—just that we're all unique and there is no one-size-fits-all approach to nutrition and dieting.

There is proof that populations lived for many generations as hunters. Low-carbohydrate diets were typical for Native Americans hunting in the plains, and the Inuit people thrive on a traditional diet practically free of carbohydrates.[2] There are also reports of Europeans crossing over to live within these hunting societies without experiencing nutritional deficiencies.[3] Whether intentional or not, carbohydrate restriction is something we as a species are capable of handling. And, as you can see, ketogenic diet patterns have been around for a long time.

Keto in Medicine

One of the most commonly known uses of ketogenic diets is for the treatment of pediatric epilepsy. In the early 1900s, Harvard Medical School researchers reported improvements in seizure control after fasting due to a change in the metabolism. It was found that the absence of food, specifically carbohydrates, forced the body to utilize fat for energy. In the 1920s, the ketogenic diet originated to treat seizures; the goal was to achieve ketosis without causing malnutrition. The diet is still used in seizure management to this day, particularly in children who do not respond to modern pharmaceutical treatments.[4]

Studies have shown that elevated ketones can also provide neurologic benefits outside the scope of epilepsy. These potential cognitive benefits have increased interest in ketone therapy for stroke rehabilitation and neurologic disorders such as Alzheimer's disease. Alzheimer's disease, now also called "type 3 diabetes," is a brain impairment linked to glucose-resistant brain cells. If brain cells are unable to uptake glucose, the simple sugar that most of our body's cells prefer as fuel, an alternative fuel is required. The heart of this therapeutic strategy is that ketones feed the impaired brain cells. In *The Alzheimer's Antidote*, certified nutrition specialist Amy Berger explains, "the brain's uptake and use of ketones is supply driven: the higher the ketones, the more the brain will take them in and use them."[5] Patients must ensure adequate ketones are available to fuel the brain with high dietary fat intake, decreased carbs, and possible ketone supplementation.[6]

Many people suffering from type 2 diabetes and other forms of clinically diagnosed insulin resistance have had success managing their illnesses with reduced carbohydrate intake. The decreased carb intake results in significantly lower blood glucose levels. This improvement in glycemic control and insulin sensitivity has made low-carb ketogenic diets an increasingly accepted approach to reversing type 2 diabetes.[7]

As you can see, the approach varies by medical necessity and desired outcomes. The diabetic looking to regulate their blood sugar has different goals and needs than the Alzheimer's patient who is aiming to fuel impaired brain cells with ketones.

Though I know it may seem obvious, I point out this distinction because many people mistakenly attempt protocols designed to address medical needs that do not align with their own goals and personal context. If you've witnessed folks taking ketone supplements or guzzling high-calorie elixirs made of butter and oils with reckless abandon in an effort to lose weight, you know exactly what I'm talking about. These dieters may have adopted a practice that supports a completely different objective without even knowing how detrimental it may be to their efforts.

Popular Low-Carb Diets

Diet fads come and go, but low-carb diets have been steadily holding their ground in the weight loss realm since the nineteenth century. In 1863, William Banting published a letter to the public describing the diet he followed to lose approximately 1 pound (454 g) per week, for a total loss of 46 pounds (21 kg). His famous "Letter on Corpulence" outlined a regimen filled with meat, fish, fruit, and vegetables while limiting the intake of carbohydrates, especially those of a starchy or sugary nature.[8]

In a move that brought ketogenic diets into the limelight, Dr. Robert C. Atkins published the popular book *Dr. Atkins' Diet Revolution* in 1972 and the follow-up title, *Atkins for Life*, in 2003. The first phase of the Atkins diet focused on achieving nutritional ketosis through carb restriction, limiting daily carbohydrate intake to 20 grams during the first two weeks. The Atkins approach slowly reincorporates carbohydrates into the diet during the following phases as the dieter progresses toward their goal weight.[9]

The paleo diet rose in popularity after Dr. Loren Cordain published *The Paleo Diet* in 2002. This plan's concept centers on the evolutionary basis for optimal human nutrition, tapping into the diets of our ancestors to guide our food choices. Cordain argues that because modern-day people have the same basic physiology as Paleolithic people, who were hunter-gatherers, we should eat a similar diet. His plan promotes the concept of feeding our bodies the foods we evolved initially to eat, rather than the staples of today's menu. As such, dairy, cereals, grains, refined sugars, and processed foods are prohibited, while carbohydrates are to come from only nonstarchy fruits and vegetables.[10]

There are a variety of other low-carb diets: the Zone Diet, Protein Power, the South Beach Diet, and Whole30, to name a few. Each is typically laid out with different guidelines and a protocol of rigid rules to follow. People have had great results following any one of the plans mentioned, but there is a core theme tying these diets together: whole food ingredients and lower carbohydrate intake than the standard American diet. They may differ in execution, but the guiding principles remain the same.

How Is Keto Different from Other Low-Carb Diets?

The primary difference between the vast number of low-carb diets and ketogenic diets is the severity of carbohydrate restriction. Not all low-carb diets are designed to induce nutritional ketosis. Just ensuring that your carb intake is lower than the standard American diet doesn't mean you will reach ketosis. Certain low-carb plans allow for much higher carb intakes than keto diets. Some don't even have restrictions on overall consumption as long as you choose the lower-carb food options when you eat.

If low-carb diets are lined up along a carbohydrate spectrum, keto falls in the lowest portion of the range. Remember, ketosis is more of a metabolic state than a diet; therefore, keto diets tend to focus on sourcing the appropriate nutrients that will support this metabolic state. Ketogenic diets are oriented toward mimicking the benefits of fasting while still eating tasty foods.

Now let's peek at the variety of ketogenic diets and see where to focus our efforts.

Types of Ketogenic Diets: Pathways to Ketosis

There are many ketogenic protocols floating around, but the one common denominator among them is carbohydrate restriction. Keep in mind that it's not the amount of fat you eat that makes a ketogenic diet; it's the limitation of carbs.

Fasting and Starvation

Ketosis can be achieved by eating nothing at all. Extended fasting or starvation leads to a metabolic state of ketosis due to the carbohydrate restriction. Most of us already know that starving is not desirable by any stretch of the imagination. In addition to severe health consequences, your body composition suffers.

When fasting, it's not just carbohydrates taken away as a fuel source; it is everything else, too. Zero energy intake. Without food intake, your body is forced to burn away its fat stores and lean body mass to survive. Lean body mass consists of everything else that makes up your body aside from adipose tissue—your muscles, organs, bones, skin, hair, and so on—that gets degraded over time during extended fasts due to the constant protein turnover in our bodies.

Without food, your body deteriorates. This is not an approach to ketosis that we will entertain in this book. Not only is this an unhealthy path, but if you do this over long enough periods of time you will become seriously ill, or worse. I don't want that, you don't want that; let's move on. Seriously.

How Does Keto Compare to Other Diets?

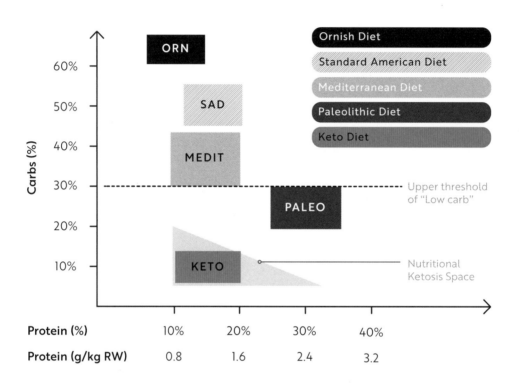

Optimal fat loss on keto requires a combination of limiting carbs, ensuring adequate protein intake, and eating energy from fat while reducing calories.

Protein-Sparing Modified Fasts

This pathway to ketosis is basically a protein-only diet. The idea behind a protein-sparing modified fast (PSMF) is that by providing the body with an adequate source of protein, you prevent the degradation of lean body mass. Muscle and other vital tissues are preserved as the body receives sufficient protein, and, by restricting both carbs and fat as energy sources, the body is forced to use stored fat for energy.

This approach is undoubtedly effective in burning body fat, but it should be approached with caution. Thoughtful supplementation and food sourcing are required—specifically to include essential fatty acids and a complete amino acid profile—to ensure the body's needs are met during a stint on one of these protocols. Typically, a PSMF is reserved for severely obese patients in clinical settings. Physique athletes may also use this diet in preparation for competitions. But, like most extreme diets, some people just use this technique to chase rapid results.[11]

Briefly, PSMF can be used as a short-term strategy, but, ultimately, it is a crash diet. It is simply not sustainable long term, and it can be challenging to adhere to. Having a couple of protein-only days here and there is not usually a problem. Lacking proper supplements and complete food sources over an extended period could cause you to get very sick or even die. Again, I'm totally serious. We will focus on the less severe, more sustainable approaches in this book.

Nutritional Ketosis for Fat Loss

Optimal fat loss on keto requires a combination of limiting carbs, ensuring adequate protein intake, and eating energy from fat while reducing calories. The body receives enough protein to prevent degradation from protein turnover, and fat is eaten for satiety and hormonal balance; a reduction in calories is factored into the mix to source adipose tissue for energy. Because carbohydrates are already minimal and protein is set to a sufficient amount to support the preservation of lean tissue, this calorie deficit comes from a reduction in dietary fat intake. This isn't nearly the dramatic decrease in calories created by eliminating all dietary fat, as is seen with a PSMF.

Nutritional ketosis for fat loss relies on a more modest deficit that allows the dieter to feel full and have plenty of food options without wreaking havoc on hormones. Most importantly, this allows the diet to be a more sustainable way of eating, which increases diet adherence. Often, this calorie deficit is intentional and tracked by dieters, but the appetite-suppressing effects of very low–carb diets can also contribute to a natural decrease in calorie intake for dieters not intentionally tracking their overall consumption. You simply don't eat as much when you're not hungry. Nutritional ketosis for fat loss is the sweet spot that will garner most of our attention throughout the remainder of this book.

Ketone Therapy and Weight Maintenance

Energy sources are fulfilled entirely through food intake. As energy needs are wholly met with diet, stored energy reserves are not burned, and body composition is maintained. That's right: no calorie restriction. For ketogenic diets used for medically therapeutic purposes revolving around high ketone levels, this is where efforts are focused. Ketone levels rise with increased fat intake, making high levels of fat consumption a top priority. Dietary fat ranges from 70 to 90 percent of total intake in diet therapies geared toward elevated ketone levels.

Ketone-based therapy relies on high ketone levels for efficacy. Patients, such as those suffering from Alzheimer's, are not using ketogenic diets to lose weight; their context is entirely different. Raised ketone levels—not a decrease in body fat—are the goal in these scenarios. See the difference?

You don't necessarily need high ketone levels to do a keto diet, especially if you are not involved in a ketone therapy for medical needs. Ketones are not the cause of fat loss; they are merely the result of fat metabolism.

Many people trying keto mistakenly follow a protocol more aligned with a medically therapeutic ketogenic diet out of simple misunderstanding or confusion about what a well-formulated high-fat diet entails. The outcome can be frustrating and unfortunate. Some dieters who head down this path don't see any change in their weight, which leads them to the conclusion that keto doesn't work. Some will actually gain weight by overdoing fat consumption, believing high fat intake is the driver behind ketogenic weight loss.

Many keto dieters are aware of the impact of calories and do lose weight while eating the very high-fat diet that aligns with ketone therapy, but the trade off comes from undereating protein to cut calories. The insufficient protein intake results in weight loss at the expense of lean tissue loss. Sure, the number on the scale goes down, but this is at the cost of your overall body composition and metabolic health. If your goal is to lose weight, it should really be to lose body fat.

Medical Ketone Therapy or Weight Maintenance

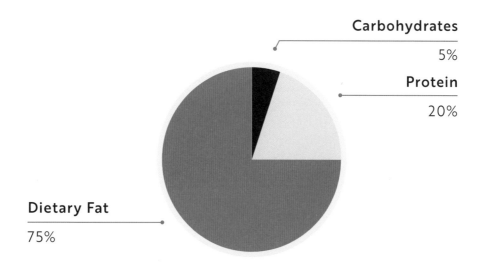

Carbohydrates
5%

Protein
20%

Dietary Fat
75%

Keto for Fat Loss

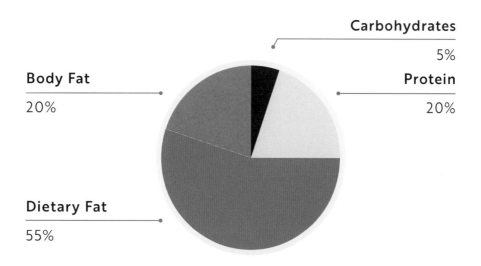

Carbohydrates
5%

Protein
20%

Body Fat
20%

Dietary Fat
55%

If you are lean or have reached your ideal weight and are committed to following a ketogenic diet, then, yes, absolutely, high-fat intake all the way. Your energy has to come from somewhere. Increasing your calories to maintenance level by upping your fat intake is indeed the route to go.

Keto for Women

Now that we have a general understanding of what keto is, we can start exploring the diet in the context of the female body. Women respond to diets differently than men, yet most dieting advice is geared toward men.

In this book, you will learn how our bodies respond to carbohydrate restriction and weight loss efforts and discover effective strategies to optimize body composition and restore hormonal imbalances. Our goal is to safely lose body fat using keto as an effective fat-burning tool—not to lose weight at all costs!

Before we jump into the actionable details, you will need a little background information to understand the basis of how the keto diet works. The fundamentals of the keto diet, including macronutrients and fat adaptation, are discussed in chapters 2 and 3. In chapters 4 through 7, you will learn the key differences for women on the keto diet, homing in on energy needs and hormones. The final chapters are all about implementation; you will learn various dieting strategies to tailor the diet to your specific needs. It may be tempting to flip to the back of the book and get started right away, but you'd be missing a lot of great information intended to clear up keto diet confusion and common misconceptions.

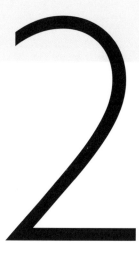

Macronutrients 101

Macronutrients—commonly referred to as "macros" in diet and nutrition circles—are the components of our food that give us energy. Think of energy, or calories, as the fuel for our bodies. Just like a car needs gas to go, the human body needs calories to support activity.

Macronutrients make up the most significant percentage of the foods we eat. They consist of carbohydrates, fat, and protein. My goal in this book is to help you determine the right balance of macronutrients to get into ketosis and recognize when adjustments are needed as your body and goals change.

Carbohydrates

This is the part of the book where I'm supposed to tell you how bad carbs are, right? Guess again, my friend. Carbohydrates are simply a type of fuel for our bodies. Rather than thinking of an entire macronutrient group (or any food, for that matter) as "good" or "bad," let's explore the effects they have on our bodies under different circumstances.

Energy from Carbs

Carbohydrates provide a major source of energy for most of the population. In the modern human diet—read: not low carb—carbohydrates supply about half the total calorie intake.

The Fate of Macronutrients during Nutritional Ketosis

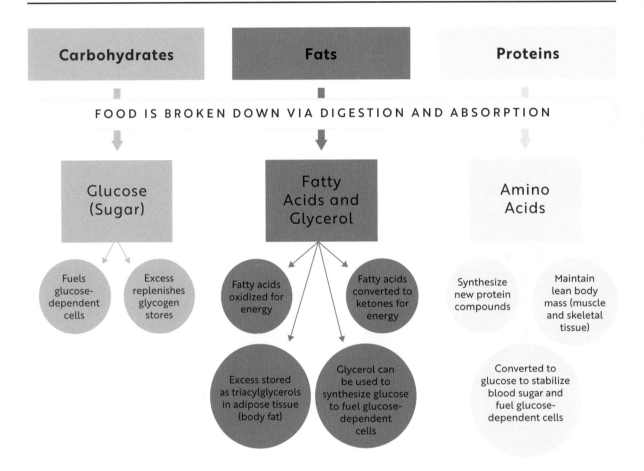

This is a far cry from a standard ketogenic diet, in which dietary carbohydrates are approximately 5 to 10 percent of total consumption.

As an energy source, carbohydrates provide 4 calories per gram. On a standard ketogenic diet, this works out to anywhere from 80 to 200 calories per day on average—not a significant source of energy by any stretch of the imagination. A standard ketogenic approach typically restricts carbohydrate intake to less than 50 grams per day.[1]

Types of Carbohydrates

Carbohydrates consist of sugar units with structures ranging from simple to complex. Simple carbs contain only one or two sugar molecules. Complex carbohydrates, as the name implies, are more elaborate and consist of many sugars bound together in chains. Most of us will recognize complex carbs by their names as they occur in our food: starch and fiber.

Our bodies can only absorb carbohydrates in their simplest form. That means complex carbs must be broken down to yield individual sugar molecules before they are accessible to the body. The more complex the carb is, the more work your body has to do to break it down. As a result, complex carbohydrates are digested and absorbed more slowly than simple sugars.

Fiber is an exception. Humans don't have digestive enzymes to break down fiber, which comes in soluble and insoluble forms. Insoluble fiber, or cellulose, passes through the digestive tract unabsorbed by the body. Although it provides a source of roughage and contributes to digestive health, it is not a source of calories. On the other hand, soluble fiber does offer a small amount of energy. Our bodies cannot digest soluble fiber, but the bacteria living in our gut can. We absorb the by-product of this process, providing approximately 2 calories per gram of soluble fiber.[2]

Where Do These Carbs Go?

Once in the blood, simple sugars are carried off to the liver for filtering. The liver traps and metabolizes some sugars, such as fructose, but most of the glucose keeps pumping through the circulatory system; this is what we know as blood sugar. The blood cycling through your body distributes glucose to tissue—such as the muscles, brain, adipose, and kidneys—where it can be taken in for energy.

As blood sugar rises, the storage hormone insulin is secreted by the pancreas. One of insulin's primary roles is to prevent blood sugar from skyrocketing after a meal. When glucose levels exceed the body's immediate needs, insulin signals cells in the muscles, liver, and fat to absorb the excess glucose. Raised levels of insulin also indirectly signal specific glucose transporters in the intestine to turn off, resulting in decreased glucose absorption. These actions help keep blood sugar stable and prevent glucose levels from getting out of control.

When the liver and muscle cells take in the excess glucose from the bloodstream, the glucose sugars bond together to form glycogen molecules. Glycogen serves as glucose storage, a reserve of energy for when the body needs it. When the demand for glucose arises, the body can quickly tap into this supply to obtain it.

Advantages of Carbohydrates

Athletic Performance Edge

Due to their quick digestion, simple sugars offer an immediate source of energy during exercise or athletic training. Strategic carbohydrate feeding is often used with athletic performance in mind.[3]

Fiber: It's Great!

Fiber enhances digestive health and plays a key role in the prevention and management of diseases. It has many beneficial properties—anti-inflammatory, anticancer, antioxidative, and antibacterial—and has been shown to improve insulin sensitivity, improve blood markers, and lower blood pressure. Slower-digesting carbohydrates, such as non-starchy vegetables and fruits, are often rich in fiber. Both the World Health Organization and Food and Agriculture Organization of the United Nations endorse a daily intake of at least 25 grams.[4]

What about Veggies and Fruits?

Fruits and vegetables, while relatively high in carbs, are important sources of micronutrients and phytochemicals. They provide a plethora of vitamins, minerals, and other phytonutrients that are beneficial to overall health and nutrition.

Disadvantages of Carbohydrates

Refined Carbohydrates and Added Sugars

Refined carbohydrates are starches that have been significantly processed to remove the bran and germ of grains. This strips them of fiber, making them quicker to digest. Vitamins, minerals, and antioxidants are also removed in the process. As a result, refined carbohydrates can cause huge surges in blood glucose while providing very little nutritional value. If you've ever heard the phrase "empty calories," refined carbohydrates certainly fill the bill. More and more food products are being made from these poor-quality carbohydrates. Americans' energy intake has increased by more than 500 calories per day compared to that at the beginning of the twentieth century, and most of those come primarily in the form of refined carbs. This substantial increase in the consumption of refined carbohydrates correlates with a simultaneous increase in insulin resistance, type 2 diabetes, and obesity.[5]

Processed food also comes loaded with added sugars, which can lead to an excess intake. The average person working a desk job doesn't have the same needs as an athlete. The quick digestion of carbs is of little use if you are sitting at a desk all day, regularly skipping the gym, and binge-watching Netflix in your spare time. Instead, they lead to repeat bouts of blood sugar spikes and crashes. When most meals or snacks consist of processed food made of refined carbohydrates and added sugars, this may lead to chronically high levels of blood sugar and insulin and contribute to insulin resistance.[6]

Insulin Resistance: It's Everywhere

Insulin resistance is when the body's cells no longer respond to the effects of the insulin hormone. Insulin's job is to cue the uptake of glucose into cells and slow glucose absorption in the intestines. In an insulin-resistant individual, however, glucose continues to flow freely into the bloodstream.[7] Glucose levels soar, and, as a result, more and more insulin is needed to trigger the intended response. As glucose concentrations remain high, the pancreas works overtime to produce enough insulin to keep the blood sugar in a healthy range. Once the pancreas can no longer keep up with the demand, the extra sugar stays in the blood. Eventually, this chronic high blood sugar can lead to type 2 diabetes, which accounts for 95 percent of all diagnosed cases of diabetes in the United States.[8]

Contributing Factors to Insulin Resistance

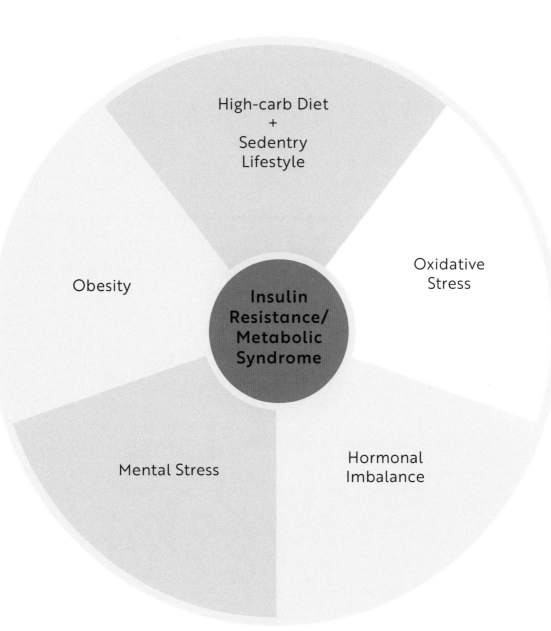

Insulin resistance is surprisingly common: According to a 2017 report by the Centers for Disease Control and Prevention, approximately one-third of the adult population in the United States has prediabetic insulin resistance, and nine out of ten of those people are unaware they have it.[9] The prevalence spans both sexes, though studies have shown that weight loss actually improves insulin resistance more in women than in men.[10] Good news for us!

Keto: Not Enough Carbs?

Now that we've talked about what happens when you eat too many carbs, you may be wondering what happens when you eat too few. If you're not continually pumping glucose into your system, won't your blood sugar get too low?

Of all the macronutrients, carbohydrates are the only ones not essential for survival. As discussed in chapter 1, nutritional ketosis allows our bodies to source energy from other nutrients in the absence of carbs. Additionally, the body can actually generate its own carbohydrates as needed, using noncarbohydrate sources. When we lack carbs in our diet, our body sources noncarb materials to synthesize glucose via a process called "gluconeogenesis." When the body demands glucose, it can produce it from within. This helps with blood sugar regulation and provides energy to glucose-dependent cells during nutritional ketosis.

Fat

Fat has been one of the most demonized nutrients throughout the twentieth and twenty-first centuries. Removing fat from food creates a void—lack of flavor, texture, nutrients—that food manufacturers often fill with sugar, refined carbohydrates, and artificial additives. It's a terrible trade-off; despite the opposite intentions, swapping fats for carbs has contributed to unprecedented levels of obesity, diabetes, and other metabolic issues. And for what? Fat doesn't have a personal vendetta against you. It isn't plotting ways to secretly expand your waistline, clog your arteries, or steal your partner. It is simply a fuel source.

Energy from Fat

If you're cutting carbohydrates with a keto diet, you need to replace that lost energy with something else. This is where the "high fat" notion in ketogenic diets comes into play.

Fat has 9 calories per gram. How much fat you eat on a ketogenic diet will depend on your body's energy requirements and your personal goals. Bear in mind: If your goal is fat loss, some of this fat energy comes served on a plate, while some will come directly from your body. Keto isn't an excuse to start eating sticks of butter.

Types of Fats

Fat is fundamental to our bodies. The most obvious form, body fat, acts as stored energy, protection for internal organs, and heat insulation. Fat also makes hormones and other

Despite the opposite intentions, swapping fats for carbs has contributed to unprecedented levels of obesity, diabetes, and other metabolic issues.

molecules and structures that are essential to our health and well-being. The fats that are most prominent in our diet are fatty acids and triacylglycerols.

Fatty acids are the most basic forms of fat and serve as the primary building blocks of triacylglycerol molecules, both in our bodies and in the food we eat. Triacylglycerols make up a huge source of energy; they are responsible for roughly 95 percent of dietary fat intake and, essentially, all stored body fat.[11] These are the types of fats that have designations such as saturated, monounsaturated, and polyunsaturated. Saturated fats are solid at room temperature—think lard, butter, or bacon grease after it cools. Unsaturated fats, like most oils, are liquid at room temperature.

Of note are two essential fatty acids the body is unable to manufacture and must obtain from the diet: linoleic acid, an omega-6 fatty acid, and alpha-linolenic acid, an omega-3 fatty acid. Both fall in the polyunsaturated category. Omega-3 fatty acids have known anti-inflammatory effects and can lower blood triglycerides.[12]

Although most energy is acquired from fatty acids during ketosis, certain cells—including nervous tissue and brain cells—are unable to use fatty acids for fuel. To get energy to these tissues, the liver converts a portion of fatty acids into ketone bodies. Important ketones include acetoacetate and β-hydroxybutyrate, which serve as crucial substitutes for glucose during carb-restricted diets or fasting.[13]

Where Do These Fats Go?
Fat digestion is focused on breaking down what we eat into small enough molecules for the body to absorb. The smaller fatty acid chains, such as medium-chain triacylglycerols, are more quickly digested and absorbed for energy. Long-chain fatty acids make up most of our dietary fat intake, and they require more digestive effort and time for the body to absorb them fully for energy.

Undigested fat slows how quickly the stomach empties, which extends the effect of the hormones involved in feeling full; this is one reason fats tend to be so sating to hunger.

In the blood, free fatty acids and other fat molecules are shuttled throughout the body and dropped off at muscle and adipose tissue to be used as energy or stored. A portion of free fatty acids are supplied to the liver and converted into ketone bodies, a process that ramps up significantly when carbohydrate intake is restricted. Ketones are released into the blood and carried to cells throughout the body for energy use.

Fat Storage

If the amount of fat consumed in a meal exceeds immediate energy demands, the body places it in storage for later use. The insulin hormone plays a role in fat storage by signaling adipose cells to take up free fatty acids and inhibiting the breakdown of stored fat. In the adipose cell, free fatty acids are synthesized into triacylglycerols, the highly concentrated stored form of energy that makes up most of our body fat.

Triacylglycerols are made up of one glycerol molecule and three fatty acid molecules bound together. When triacylglycerols in adipose tissue are needed for fuel, the fatty acids are split off from glycerol and released back into the blood, where they are then transported to various tissues throughout the body to be used for fuel. In a calorie deficit, this is how body fat is burned.

Too Little Fat

If you are restricting carbohydrates, your predominant source of energy is fat. Cutting both carbohydrates and fats creates an unsustainable calorie deficit for the average dieter. A very lean person could not survive on a diet low in both carbs and fat, as there would be minimal stored fuel left to burn and provide energy.

Fatty Acid Deficiency

There are two essential fatty acids in the diet that the body cannot synthesize: linoleic acid and alpha-linolenic acid. Without enough of these in the diet, a condition known as fatty acid deficiency can occur. This is typically seen in individuals who are receiving parenteral nutrition (i.e., feeding nutrients through an IV) or who have fat malabsorption issues; however, it can develop with extremely low-fat or no-fat diets. Symptoms of fatty acid deficiency include rough, scaly skin, dermatitis, impaired wound healing, and other nutrient deficiencies. Lack of essential fatty acids can also influence cell signaling and gene expression.[14]

Nutrient Deficiencies

Many vitamins critical for health are fat soluble, meaning they are absorbed in fats and oils. Vitamins A, D, E, and K are all fat soluble and are carried into the body along with fats obtained in the diet during the digestive process. Without adequate fat in the diet, vitamin absorption is affected, and deficiencies in vitamins A, D, E, and K may develop.[15]

Too Much Fat

Is overdoing it on fat possible during the keto diet? Absolutely. A resounding yes. Even with limited carb intake and adequate protein, excess fat that you take in will accumulate as stored body fat. If you are overeating while on a ketogenic diet, it is not just possible but highly likely you will gain body fat. Many people mistakenly believe that just because their carbohydrate intake is low, they can eat unlimited amounts of fat. Sadly, this is not the case; overeating fat beyond your energy needs, even in ketosis, will result in fat gains. The fat that is unable to be used for energy will be stored in adipose tissue; regularly eating above caloric needs results in a stockpile of stored energy.

Omega-6 versus Omega-3 Fatty Acids

While both are critical for growth and repair, omega-6 fatty acids and omega-3 fatty acids compete with each other in the body. Fighting for enzymes to drive important chemical reactions in the body, omega-6 tends to outcompete omega-3 due to an imbalanced ratio favoring omega-6.[16] Most people get plenty of omega-6 fatty acids in their diet without even trying but struggle to achieve the minimal amount of omega-3 needed to keep the body running in an optimal state. Overconsumption of foods high in omega-6 can be inflammatory to the body and has been implicated in a variety of pathological conditions, including metabolic syndrome, insulin resistance, Alzheimer's, and asthma.[17] Limiting omega-6 intake and increasing foods rich in omega-3–can help combat the common imbalance and increase the anti-inflammatory omega-3 fatty acid concentration.[18]

Protein

Protein is not an energy source in the traditional sense. Instead, it supplies the fundamental pieces to build various components of our bodies. In the absence of carbohydrates, protein intake is even more critical.[19]

Energy from Protein

While protein provides 4 calories per gram, its primary function is not to provide fuel for the body; it is to build the body and the components that make it function.

The amount of protein you eat will vary based on your body composition and activity levels. Adequate protein intake recommended for a standard ketogenic diet ranges from 0.6 to 1.0 gram per 1 pound (454 g) of lean body mass.[20]

Although keto is not necessarily a high-protein diet, it may seem like it is when you're cutting back on your dietary fat intake to burn body fat. In a Diet Doctor interview (2011), Dr. Stephen Phinney explained how the diet may appear misleadingly high in protein during fat loss stages.

Protein Turnover

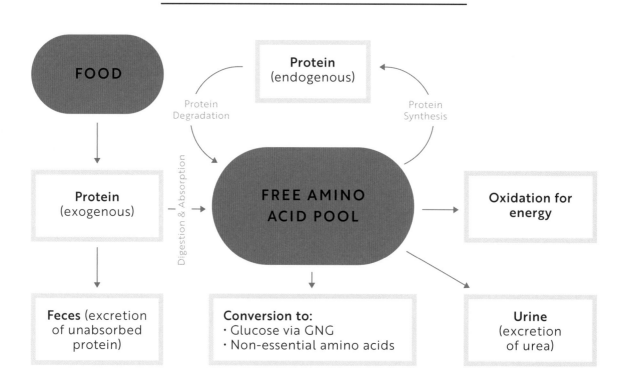

Somebody who intends to lose weight might eat 1,400 calories per day but [burn] twice as many calories per day. A heavy male might burn 2,800 calories a day. The rest—the other half—is coming from body fat. So, when you look at what that person eats, what's on the plate, if that person is eating 1,400 calories and 600 to 800 calories of that comes from protein, that looks like that's a half-protein diet. So, it looks high protein. But that's only what the mouth sees. What the body is seeing is a moderate protein intake because the mouth isn't seeing that half that's coming from inside.

But once you get to maintenance—maintenance means you're not burning any more body fat. And that requires that all of the fat that you are burning each day . . . has to come from the outside.

—Dr. Stephen Phinney, author of *The Art and Science of Low Carbohydrate Living* and *The Art and Science of Low Carbohydrate Performance*

During nutritional ketosis, sufficient amounts of protein are required to the support body tissues, glucose production, and other biological activities, while body-fat stores are used to supply the high-fat energy requirements.

Types of Proteins
Proteins are the building blocks of the body. In fact, the body tissues themselves are made up of proteins; they offer structural support and provide strength and shape to skin, tendons, membranes, muscles, and bones. As enzymes, proteins are biological catalysts that facilitate chemical reactions in the body. Some hormones, such as insulin, are proteins that regulate processes in the body. Proteins help keep the body in balance by regulating fluid and acidity. Transporter proteins are responsible for carrying substances such as vitamins, minerals, and oxygen to their destinations around the body. Antibodies are made of proteins; they protect the body against diseases by inactivating foreign invaders. While proteins do provide some fuel and glucose as needed for the body's energy needs, proteins are responsible for a whole lot more than that!

Amino acids are the building blocks of proteins, and twenty different amino acids make up the extensive collection of protein structures. Think of amino acids as a set of LEGOS. These pieces can build any number of things: castles, space shuttles, dragons. These structures can also be broken back down into individual bricks and rebuilt into other things: trains, robots, helicopters. When you eat protein, the same thing happens. The turkey breast or steak gets disassembled into individual amino acids by the body, then reconstructed into the form of protein your body needs—muscle tissue, hormones, enzymes, antibodies, and so on.[21]

Essential amino acids are the building blocks that your body is unable to manufacture from within and must be collected from the diet. This is one reason protein consumption is so

MACRONUTRIENT OVERVIEW			
	Carbohydrates	**Fat**	**Protein**
Calories (per gram)	4*	9	4
Primary Role	Energy	Energy	Building components of body
Primary Form in Food	Sugar Starches Fiber	Triacylglycerols	Protein
Building Blocks (Subunits)	Sugars	Fatty acids	Amino acids
Stored As	Glycogen in liver and muscles	Triacylglycerols in adipose tissue	n/a
Slow Digestion	**Complex carbs:** Starches Fiber	Long-chain fatty acids (MCTs)	Essential amino acids absorbed slightly quicker
Quick Digestion	Simple sugars Refined carbs	Short- and medium-chain fatty acids (MCTs)	Essential amino acids absorbed slightly quicker
Satiety Level	Low**	High	Highest
High-Quality Sources	Fibrous veggies Fibrous fruits	Monounsaturated Polyunsaturated omega-3 Saturated	Complete amino acid profiles; mainly animal sources
Low-Quality Sources	Refined carbs Simple sugars	Trans fats Polyunsaturated omega-6	Incomplete amino acid profiles: mainly plant sources
Daily Intake during Ketosis	Less than 50 g	Varies	0.6 to 1.0 g/pound (454 g) lean body mass
Changes during Ketosis	No longer primary source of energy	Some free fatty acids are converted to ketones, as needed	Some amino acids are converted to glucose, as needed

* Insoluble fiber = 0 calories/gram; soluble fiber = 2 calories/gram
** Fiber is an exception that provides high satiety.

important—without a complete set of amino acids your body runs the risk of not being able to make the proteins it needs. If half of your LEGO pieces are missing, you are limited by more than just your imagination.

Where Do These Proteins Go?

The liver is the primary site for uptake of most amino acids following ingestion of a protein-containing meal, though other organs take some in as well. The liver monitors the concentration of amino acids, adjusting amino acid breakdown and synthesis according to the needs of the body.

The body doesn't store proteins for later use. As protein is degraded into amino acids, some can be recycled by the body for new purposes, and others are excreted as waste. Thus, adequate protein intake is critical to provide a steady stream of new amino acids to balance the cycle.

Too Little Protein

When amino acid quantities are low, protein degradation increases and protein production is inhibited. Protein breakdown occurs throughout the body, but due to the relative size and mass of muscles compared to other tissues, breakdown within muscles accounts for 25 to 35 percent of total protein turnover.[22] Muscle tissue is not repaired, and loss of lean body mass often results. Additionally, various forms of malnutrition may occur without complete amino acid sources.

While the recommended daily allowance (RDA) for adults is 0.8 grams per kilogram of body weight per day, it has been repeatedly argued that the current RDA is inadequate for the average person.[23] The RDA also becomes insufficient during periods of energy restriction, such as dieting for weight loss.[24] Again, the RDA falls short when it comes to athletic training, as it is unable to support new muscle protein synthesis, repair to muscle damage, or maintenance of lean mass in individuals involved in sports, training, or strenuous exercise.[25]

During nutritional ketosis, the body manufactures glucose from noncarbohydrate sources to maintain blood sugar and support glucose-dependent cells. Amino acids are included in these noncarbohydrate sources. As such, nutritional ketosis increases the body's demand for amino acids; if they are not supplied in adequate amounts from the diet, the body will source amino acids for gluconeogenesis from tissue throughout the body.

Too Much Protein

Of all the macronutrients, protein provides the highest satiety,[26] making overeating it challenging. Very high protein intakes are typically achieved through both diet and supplementation; however, there are no upper intake levels established for protein at this time.[27]

Though reports of adverse consequences from very high protein intake do exist, they have been deemed insufficient to warrant recommended limits, with little evidence supporting health risks.[28]

However, there is no real benefit to overeating protein beyond your body's demands. Overfeeding on protein can be a strategy to build lean body mass, but this is only effective when paired with sports or resistance training, which increases the body's underlying need for the nutrient.[29]

Gluconeogenesis: The GNG Controversy

We know that the body can make glucose from amino acids. A common concern for keto dieters is the notion that when extra protein is eaten, the amino acids are immediately converted to glucose and—poof!—you will no longer be in ketosis. That's not really how our bodies work, though. This is an ill-conceived idea based on the assumption that just because the body *can* turn amino acids into glucose, it *will*. The body dictates what happens to the amino acids based on biological demand. Some will be used for tissue repair, others for hormones, some will even be turned into ketones, and yes—when the body needs it—some will be turned into glucose. This theory also assumes the body producing glucose is detrimental to your diet, when, in reality, we need this source of glucose to support glucose-dependent cells and keep blood sugar stable.[30] Gluconeogenesis isn't bad; it's totally natural and necessary under ketogenic conditions.

If that's not enough to get you feeling good about gluconeogenesis, what if I told you it makes your body burn more calories? During carbohydrate restriction, the increased gluconeogenesis that occurs results in an increase in energy expenditure.[31] A boost in your metabolism is certainly good news for those trying to lose weight and improve body composition.

Patients with a medical need for high ketone levels (Alzheimer's, epilepsy, etc.) may have cause for concern that excess amino acids turn into glucose, spike insulin, and drive down ketones;[32] however, the average dieter doesn't need to worry about ketone levels. Don't short-change yourself on protein for fear of something that doesn't apply to you. In my experience, people on ketogenic diets are so wrapped up with the idea of eating "too much" protein they often don't get enough. When it comes to protein, it's best to err on the higher end and ensure adequate intake.

3

The Fat-Burning Advantage

If carbs and fat are just fuel, what's so bad about combining the two? Do you really have to choose one or the other? To answer these questions, let's look at how our body responds to the high-fat, high-carb combo.

Carbs and Fat: The Perfect Storm

Foods high in both fat and carbs are rarely found in nature. When they are, they are highly prized sources of energy, fiber, and nutrients. Think nuts or avocados—fatty, fibrous, slowly digested, steady supplies of energy. As former hunter-gatherers, we are wired to covet these rare combos. Today, however, we don't have to look far for high-carb, high-fat foods—we just need to visit our nearest convenience store. If you cruise by the drive-thru, you don't even have to get out of your car to get them!

Of course, these are not nourishing powerhouses; they are overly processed refined carbo-hydrates, sugars, and fats, all conveniently packaged for quick consumption. This high-carb, high-fat combo forms the basis of what we now know as the standard American diet.[1] It's a recipe for overconsumption and fat storage.

A Powerful Reward System: It Feels So Good!

When we eat food, our body's chemical messengers fire up and communicate with our systems in various ways. Certain neurotransmitters, the chemical messengers of the brain, are triggered by particular nutrients and food combinations. Dopamine is the neurotransmitter tied to our internal reward center. When we eat carbs or fat, dopamine surges occur through one of two distinct pathways. When we eat carbs and fat together, both pathways ignite, which amplifies the perceived reward. Think of it like this: If the reward for eating carbs was a compliment, and the reward for eating fat was a backrub, eating carbs and fat together would be like winning a Woman of the Year award while being pampered at a luxury spa. The brain perceives an exaggerated megareward when we eat high-carb, high-fat meals.[2]

This ties in to the intrinsic value we place on foods high in both fat and carbs. Calorie to calorie, high-carb, high-fat food combos are simply more valuable to people than their single-macronutrient counterparts. Studies have shown that when matched for calories, people are willing to pay more of their hard-earned cash for foods with a high-fat, high-carb macronutrient composition than those with just high carbs or high fats;[3] they're simply worth more to us.

Serotonin is another neurotransmitter affected by food intake. When we eat carbohydrates, serotonin levels change and appetite increases.[4] When dopamine and serotonin overlap, our drive to eat expands beyond our basic hunger levels. These types of rewards and positive feedback influence our eating behaviors over time. This leads to snacking when we aren't even hungry, eating more even when we're full, and reaching for the feel-good food instead of the healthy choices.

Increased Fat Storage

As your blood glucose increases after you eat carbs, your insulin rises to drive those blood sugars into storage. And insulin is responsible for mediating fat storage as well. If you're eating carbs and fat in excess (as is often the case with these ultrarewarding food combos), the fat in your food is being guided to your adipose tissue reserves. Now imagine what happens if most meals are built around carbs and fat. The fat storage will quickly fill up and expand, driving weight gain and sabotaging body composition.

When you eat food low in carbs but rich in other macronutrients, such as protein and fats, the insulin response is not nearly as dramatic. The insulin hormone is not automatically primed for fat storage in these scenarios, which can help you maintain weight or access fat stores for energy to lose body fat.

You Have to Choose

The first step in dealing with the high-carb, high-fat dilemma is simply acknowledging it is a problem—one affecting all of us, everywhere. Overeating has never been easier or more convenient. And, as a society, we have never been fatter.

The second step: Take action and break the cycle. Choose carbs or choose fat, but stop choosing both at the same time. Your health will thank you.

Choosing Fat: Becoming a Fat-Burner

Choosing fat as your leading fuel source has its advantages. For those primarily interested in fat loss and improvements in body composition, the chief benefit comes from being more efficient at burning fat for fuel, both from dietary sources and from your body. On a standard ketogenic diet, insulin levels will be kept at bay, allowing easy access to fat reserves. For women, this can be a hugely beneficial way to modify our innate biology.

Ketosis versus Fat Adaptation

Here's what to expect as your body adapts to a low-carb ketogenic diet.

Getting Into Ketosis (2 to 3 days)

Becoming a fat-burner doesn't just happen. There is a brief adjustment period as your body metabolizes its remaining carbs, which is what we in the biz call "getting into ketosis." This usually only takes a few days.

Nutritional ketosis occurs soon after restricting carbohydrate intake. As carbs are limited, the body begins burning through its glycogen stores to supply cells with their preferred fuel—glucose—which rapidly depletes the stored carb energy within the body. Glycogen stores in the liver and muscle tissue are depleted within a couple of days, though physical activity can speed the process. Once this stored glucose energy is used up, the body is forced to start making ketones from fatty acids and manufacturing its own glucose to replace what is no longer supplied through diet.

Men versus Women: Who Stores It Better?

When it comes to fat storage, the female body stockpiles fat like that's its job. From an evolutionary standpoint, you could argue that it is. After all, the survival of a species depends on its reproductive success. Though it may not be relevant to your personal interests, the female body is designed to support the extremely costly process of growing, carrying, and nourishing offspring. This process requires large amounts of energy, so our bodies become really good at storing it. The female body favors adipose tissue storage and resists the loss of energy stores, even during long periods of food scarcity.[5]

Increased energy storage was a fantastic evolutionary strategy when access to food was feast or famine—our survival as a species depended on it! We were able to stay alive, reproduce, and protect our offspring when food was unavailable. In today's climate, this innate survival mechanism is a double-edged sword. Now that we have an overabundance of highly palatable, high-calorie food at our disposal, unwanted weight gain is a snap and losing body fat proves to be an uphill battle.

The obesity epidemic affects both sexes, but women are at a fundamental disadvantage when it comes to excess body fat. Women typically have twice the amount of body fat as men, and our bodies don't burn it as readily as theirs do. At rest and in the postabsorptive state (3 to 18 hours after a meal), female bodies actively store free fatty acids while male bodies readily burn them and mobilize energy stores.[6] By default, the female body is better at hoarding body fat and less willing to burn it for energy.

Timeline of Fat Adaptation

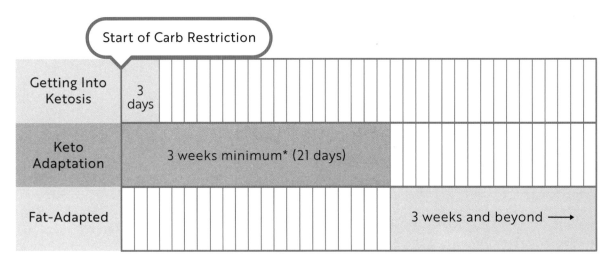

Actual timeline varies; some individuals take longer to make adaptations.

Keto-Adaptation (3 to 6 weeks)

Initially, the process of using ketones and fatty acids for fuel is inefficient. In the beginning, cells throughout the body still prefer to burn glucose. When it's available, the cells take up sugar even when ketones and fatty acids are readily accessible. At this time, the brain continues to run primarily on glucose being made from within the body.

During extended carbohydrate restriction, the body undergoes physiological adaptations similar to what occurs in extended fasts. Energy partitioning changes; the brain becomes less dependent on glucose and utilizes more ketones, muscle protein breakdown is reduced, and cells throughout the body become better at using fatty acids and ketones for energy.

This is an adjustment period known as keto adaptation or fat adaptation. Specifically, this references the body's shift to using fat as the primary energy source during rest, activity, and exercise.[7]

If carbohydrates are eaten during this time, the body will default to its routine metabolism, and ketone production will decrease until carbs are restricted again. This only prolongs the time it takes the body to adapt. If significant carbohydrate fuel continues to be introduced

ENERGY EXCHANGE AND CONSUMPTION		
Fuel Used by Brain	**Week 1**	**Week 6**
Glucose	↑	↓
Ketones	↓	↑
Reserved Fuel Use	**Week 1**	**Week 6**
Adipose tissue	↓	↑
Muscle and liver glycogen stores	↑	↓
Muscle protein degradation	↑	↓

This table provides a summary of the energy usage adaptations that develop during extended carb restriction.

in your diet, the body will not have any reason to modify its preferred fuel source. Though the time required varies from person to person, this process usually takes a minimum of three weeks.[8]

Think about when you travel to work. There is a typical route you take to get from point A to point B. One day, you discover the road you take to get to your job is closed, a detour sign has been posted, and traffic has been rerouted in another direction. The first day, this comes as a surprise to commuters and traffic slows as drivers assess alternate navigation to their destinations. With each passing day the road continues to be closed, commuters become more familiar with their alternate routes and navigate the closure more efficiently. It may not be the fastest route, but it's the best way to go given the circumstances. Think about the shifting metabolic pathways that occur during ketogenic diets as traffic detours; at first, they aren't efficient, but over time, you adjust and adapt accordingly.

Fat Adaptation (6 weeks and beyond)
Once your body has fully acclimated to your low-carb ketogenic diet, you are fully fat-adapted. Congratulations! You made it! You're a fat-burner now! This means the cells in your body have made the necessary adaptations to preferentially burn fatty acids and ketones for fuel instead of glucose. There will always be glucose-dependent cells running exclusively on sugar made within the body; however, the predominant and favored fuel sources in this state are mostly fat. Efficient, accelerated fat burning—huzzah!

What happens if you eat carbs now? A carb excursion in a fat-adapted body won't completely derail the metabolic adaptations the body has achieved. At this point, you can intermittently eat carbohydrates and easily dip in and out of nutritional ketosis without having to start the acclimation process all over again. When your body has fully made adaptations to a ketogenic diet, your metabolism has changed. So, as long as you keep your carb intake low *most of the time*, you can still reap the benefits of being fat-adapted, i.e., burning fat as the primary fuel source. Many people following standard ketogenic diets never reintroduce carbohydrates into the diet, and that's perfectly fine. But this ability to switch back and forth between fuel sources quickly allows for strategic use of carbohydrates in those who feel they could benefit. Whether it is an athletic-related carb feeding or a sweet treat on a special occasion, periodic carbs have less effect on your overall fat-burning abilities once the body has become fat-adapted. Once the carbs are metabolized, you're back to burning fat!

Being fat-adapted also affords the flexibility of increasing your carbohydrate intake a bit higher than necessary for a standard ketogenic diet—you may not be in ketosis once you do this, but you'll still be burning fat. For people who don't necessarily need, or want, to live in a perpetual state of nutritional ketosis, this can be relieving news to hear after all the effort you've gone through to modify your diet.

While eating carbs won't immediately undo these adaptations, your body will return to preferentially burning sugar when carb intake is high for an extended period. Just as we were able to become fat-burners by changing our dietary intake over time, we can renew our sugar-burner membership as well. If you choose to become a fat-burner once again, strict carbohydrate restriction is required to achieve the metabolic fat-burning adaptations.

Benefits of Keto Adaptation for Women

A bangin' bod is easy to see, but that's not where the ball stops rolling. Let's take a look at some other benefits of keto-adaption beyond weight loss.

Improved Body Composition

The ketogenic edge often lies in the superior fat-burning abilities that contribute to improved body composition. Not only does the body become better at using fat for energy, but ketogenic diets are protein-sparing, meaning muscle breakdown is conserved. When combined with adequate protein intake, being keto-adapted puts the body at a unique advantage: You can lose body fat while preserving muscle. It's the ideal weight loss scenario.

How many diets have you judged purely by a declining number on the scale? Most diet programs focus on overall weight loss without regard for your precious lean body mass. Just because the number on the scale is dropping doesn't mean you are losing fat! On the other hand, nutritional ketosis allows for increased fat oxidation while keeping your muscles shapely and other lean tissue safe.

Amazing Appetite Control and Dietary Compliance

Do you think of the word *diet* and immediately imagine endless days of hunger and deprivation? Luckily, a well-known side effect of nutritional ketosis is decreased appetite. During the first few days of limiting carbohydrates, cravings and hunger pangs may rear their ugly heads, but once the body has fully adapted to burning fat for fuel, many people report these symptoms all but disappear. Ketogenic diets are notorious for their effective appetite suppression and hunger control.[12] Studies have shown that during traditional diets, hunger increases as weight is lost; however, when carbohydrates are restricted with weight loss, the apparent increase in hunger is absent.[13]

Ketosis versus Ketoacidosis

Nutritional ketosis is a perfectly normal shift in metabolism. However, when people hear the words "ketosis," they often confuse it with "ketoacidosis," a life-threatening complication that can occur with type 1 diabetes mellitus related to insulin deficiency. Ketoacidosis results in dangerously high blood glucose, an excessive accumulation of ketone bodies, and plasma pH drops resulting in an acidic shift in the blood.[10]

Though the names sound similar, ketosis and ketoacidosis are two completely different things. The critical difference boils down to whether the metabolic state is protective or toxic. During a ketogenic diet, nutritional ketosis produces ketones that offer neuroprotection as energy substrates, chemical signaling, and regulation of gene expression. It's all good. A diabetic ketoacidosis episode is neurotoxic and damaging to the brain cells.[11]

Reduced hunger and improved appetite control can certainly make following a ketogenic diet easier to adhere to, particularly during weight loss efforts. If you change your way of eating only to be constantly plagued by hunger, there's a slim chance you'll last long. However, if you change your way of eating and can consistently eat less because your body is actively signaling you to do so, you've found a recipe for successful weight loss. If there's one thing everyone can agree on, it is that the most effective diet is the one you stick with.

Alternative Metabolic Pathways: Healing Without Prescriptions

Although this book isn't geared toward medical uses of ketogenic diets, I would be remiss not to include the possible therapeutic benefits associated with carbohydrate restriction. There will undoubtedly be many women who read this book and find the restorative properties of ketogenic diets outweigh any of the aforementioned fat-burning benefits. After all, the food we eat directly affects our overall health and wellness, not just our outward appearance.

Insulin Resistance

For those with varying degrees of insulin resistance, ketogenic diets offer a dietary approach that minimizes the need to continuously battle against the body's faulty response to insulin. By keeping incoming carbohydrates low, the struggle to overcome elevated blood glucose with excess insulin can be avoided. For women with insulin resistance, such as type two diabetes, polycystic ovarian syndrome (PCOS), or metabolic syndrome, carb restriction may help manage symptoms commonly addressed with prescription medicine.

Curb Your Inflammation

Inflammation occurs as your body's natural defense mechanism to ward off infection or heal an injury. It's not inherently a bad thing, but chronic inflammation that frequently recurs or continues over long periods is often the root of many diseases and health conditions. Inflammation is linked to insulin resistance, cardiovascular disease, cancer, Alzheimer's, Crohn's disease, irritable bowel syndrome, arthritis, and fibromyalgia—to name just a few.

Refined carbohydrates and processed sugars increase inflammatory agents, manifesting as a number of chronic health issues.[14] By eliminating these types of foods, ketogenic diets have been shown to alleviate inflammation in a wide variety of scenarios—from tumor suppression to rheumatoid arthritis therapy.[15] In women with PCOS, the most common endocrine disorder for women of reproductive age, carbohydrate restriction has been found to attenuate the low-grade inflammation characteristic of the disorder.[16]

For those using ketogenic diets for weight loss, the calorie restriction will also have an anti-inflammatory effect. Regardless of diet composition, weight loss is a crucial factor in reducing inflammation.[17]

Better Moods and Improved Mental Health

Neurologic disorders, such as Alzheimer's, can benefit from the alternate metabolic pathways afforded by keto adaptation. In cases where brain cells are not getting the energy needed, ketogenic diets provide a way to deliver energy that may be used in different forms.

Ketogenic diets have a profound effect on multiple targets implicated in the pathophysiology of mood disorders. Studies and case reports have demonstrated antidepressant and mood-stabilizing effects from keto. New research suggests that ketogenic diets may offer functional relief for depression and bipolar disorders.[18]

The List Goes On!

Entire books have been written on the therapeutic benefits of ketogenic diets in various contexts; my review here only begins to scratch the surface. Ketogenic diets are being used for purposes ranging from fertility treatments to migraine relief, and new research is being published daily in support of choosing fat for fuel far beyond weight loss.

Avoiding Diet Dogma

Fads, dogma, and doctrine run rampant when it comes to diets. Though there is overwhelming scientific evidence supporting the efficacy of ketogenic diets for a wide range of people and purposes, low-carb communities are not void of their share of myths and misinformation.

The rise of the internet and social media has given us the ability to connect with people who share similar interests and ideologies from all over the world. People are attracted to cohesive groups as a means of defining identity and belonging, but when dietary behavior is involved, this can create "food cults" in which values, rituals, and doctrine are established.[19] Although this can provide comfort and community, it can also bring guilt, judgment, and ostracism for those who deviate from the norm.[20] Even within ketogenic communities, controversy and conflict persist regarding best practices, misinformation can be perpetuated, and individual context is often completely disregarded. It's unfortunate, but that's what happens when you get large groups of people involved with *anything*.

To address this, I'd like to point out the biggest points of contention, myths, and misinformation I've experienced over the years. Consider this a friendly heads-up and reminder to focus on your own personal context.

Myth #1: Calories Don't Exist

Yikes. To lose weight, the body must burn stored energy. To do that, the body must burn more energy than it takes in—in other words, a calorie deficit is needed. In the same vein, weight gain is caused by an overconsumption of energy—an excess calorie intake. The old adage "calories in, calories out" still rings true. Focusing exclusively on calories can be problematic for reasons covered throughout this book, but denying their role in our body composition is foolish. We'll tackle calorie needs for women in more detail in the next chapter, but this is probably the biggest misunderstanding entangled with keto diets.

Myth #2: Ketones Make You Skinny

No. Ketones are simply by-products of metabolism. When your liver converts fatty acids or amino acids to ketones, it's just to fuel cells that need energy. The mere presence of ketones is not negating your overall energy intake; they *are* energy. Ketone supplements marketed as quick and easy shortcuts to weight loss are misleading. If your body is unable to use excess ketones, they are excreted as waste in the urine and exhaled in the breath. If you end up taking ketone supplements hoping they will aid your weight loss efforts, it will end one of two ways—neither of which is conducive to fat loss:

1. You'll add extra fuel your body needs to burn through before it gets to your fat stores.
2. You'll have very expensive pee.

This is like thinking that simply adding more dietary fat will magically make you burn more body fat. And that leads me to my next point.

Myth #3: The More Fat, the Better!

Again, our body fat serves as a reserve for energy when intake is low. If we're limiting carbohydrates and eating adequate protein, the fat macronutrient is the variable that must be adjusted to access stored body fat effectively. The fat provided in our meals is fuel the body must burn before reaching the fuel stored in the fat in our bodies. Do you take money out of savings to go shopping while there's money in your checking account? Eating fat during nutritional ketosis provides energy, helps us feel full, provides a way for certain vitamins to enter the body, and helps us regulate our hormones. But adding dietary fat thinking it will somehow result in decreased body fat misses the mark entirely. Think about that the next time someone argues you need a higher fat intake to do keto effectively. Hint: It won't help.

Have you seen the growing trend to blend butter into coffee to increase the fat content? It's not actually conducive to fat loss. It is a calorically dense beverage that provides very little nutritional value. Rather than accelerating fat loss, it can have the opposite effect: Your body will be busy burning butter rather than attacking your fat stores for fuel.

Myth #4: Carbs Are Evil!

When I talk about keto, I like to try to keep the snark to a minimum. I'd like people to take me seriously, after all. But when I hear this myth, I can't keep my eyes from rolling. Carbs are not evil. Food is not good or bad; it has no moral value.

Just because we have chosen to use fat for fuel doesn't mean that people who pick carbs are wrong. Just because you are choosing fat now doesn't mean you can't elect carbs later. Just because you are on a ketogenic diet doesn't mean you have to avoid every miniscule gram of carbs.

Myth #5: That's Not Keto!

Time for a quiz:

> Is ketosis caused by eliminating gluten?
> Is ketosis caused by eliminating dairy?
> Is ketosis caused by eliminating soy?
> Is ketosis caused by eliminating peanuts?
> Is ketosis caused by eliminating foods?

The answer is no to all. So, what do these questions all have in common? Potentially inflammatory foods. Keyword: *potentially*. Armed with a general awareness that these types of foods have the capacity to cause inflammation, people often assume they must be bad for everyone and insist they don't belong in a ketogenic diet. And that's when you start to hear, "That's not keto!" However, these arguments are grounded more in personal food values and beliefs than anything related to carb restriction or ketogenic diets.[21]

Of course, many foods are potentially problematic, but blindly avoiding very specific ingredients without a tangible reason is unnecessary. Just because certain foods *can* cause issues doesn't mean they *will* cause issues—there's no point in guessing. *Her* gluten sensitivity is not *your* gluten sensitivity. Rather than assuming a set of foods is inherently detrimental, we will go through the process of identifying *your* food sensitivities later in this book. After all, your diet should make sense for you, not someone else.

If someone tips you off that something is "not keto," it tends to be reflective of their personal way of eating. Sometimes they may even misunderstand what ketosis actually is. The phrases "allowed" and "not allowed" don't really have a place in the context of ketogenic diets. You can set your own parameters on your diet, but please don't impose them on others. That's not helpful.

Now, what about known antiketogenic ingredients, such as sugars and starches? If you're reading a nutrition label and spot words such as "potato starch" or "cane sugar," should you be concerned? Are these words the official telltale sign whether something is keto or not? The answer: It depends. In minimal amounts, even antiketogenic ingredients won't affect ketosis. The quantity consumed, your activity levels, your carbohydrate tolerance, and your state of metabolism will dictate whether or not it affects ketosis. Keto isn't black and white. The gray areas can be confusing when you're just getting started, even frustrating for those who like things cut and dried. Don't stress; we will keep things as simple as possible during your transition to ensure your success.

A Diet that Lasts . . . Forever?

How long should a ketogenic diet last? It's up to you. The "best" diet is the sustainable one. Finding a healthful way of eating that aligns with your values, food preferences, and limitations is at the root of long-term dietary compliance and success.

Maintaining a healthy weight is not achieved by simply dieting for a few weeks; you aren't finished when you reach your goal weight. Getting healthy is a marathon, not a sprint. It's about creating a lifestyle that incorporates healthy eating practices and physical activity that supports an energy balance for your body.

Many people find they thrive on ketogenic diets and continue to eat low carb indefinitely. For these people, keto becomes more of a sustainable lifestyle choice than a diet with an expiration date. Returning to the same eating habits that led you to a higher-than-normal weight will bring you right back to where you started. If keto proves to support dietary habits that meet your nutritional needs and, ultimately, feels sustainable, by all means, stick with it.

If, however, nutritional ketosis proves to be a constant challenge, whatever the reason may be, don't feel sorry about incorporating carbohydrates into your diet. There are plenty of nutritious sources of carbs and healthy ways to live your life as a sugar burner. Your hard-earned progress won't immediately unravel.

Not all of you are going into this diet thinking you will stick with it indefinitely. Some people have a day or goal in mind that will signal the end of their diet. Perhaps it's a big event, such as a wedding or vacation. Maybe you've already decided to try keto for a month or two and then switch to something else. Whatever you ultimately decide, understand that a temporary stint on keto won't erase your old habits. Any way of eating you choose is going to require work to undo unhealthy eating behaviors. Permanent results require permanent lifestyle changes.

As much as I'd love to provide a magical key to the perfect one-size-fits-all diet, I can't. It doesn't exist. But what I can do is offer an effective alternative to high-carb diets, which most women have already tried and failed. Whether you decide to stick with keto for life or use the diet as a passing means to an end, I'll do my best to help you make informed food decisions and offer practical solutions to help you on your journey to better health.

FUNDAMENTALS OF THE FEMALE BODY

Moving in on more female-specific territory, this part details exactly how women's bodies respond to both diet and exercise.

Starting with the concept of energy balance, chapter 4 drives home the most fundamental component of the weight loss puzzle for women. You'll learn when a calorie deficit is appropriate, connect the dots between macronutrients and calories, and take on some of the biggest misconceptions women face while losing weight on the keto diet.

Hormonal balance is the theme of chapters 5 and 6. You will learn the incredible role your menstrual cycle (or lack of it) plays in your eating habits, metabolism, and body composition in chapter 5. The hormone discussion continues on into chapter 6, where you will learn exactly how hormones affect your metabolic rate and drive to eat, how keto can help restore balance to your hormones, and whether or not long-term carbohydrate restriction is the best choice for women.

Chapter 7 is for the fitness fanatics and anyone considering incorporating an exercise routine while doing keto. (Hint: You absolutely should!) You'll learn all about fueling your activities with fat and scenarios that may require strategic use of carbohydrates.

4

Calories:
The New "C" Word

I personally know the frustration that comes along with struggling to manage weight and being told simply to "eat less." Before a nutrition career was even a twinkle in my eye, I was a serial dieter and I had some serious ups and downs. I remember sitting in the doctor's office in tears explaining my dilemma and looking for answers: I had rapidly gained around 50 pounds (22.5 kg) on top of already being overweight, my skin was covered in acne, and I had stopped menstruating completely.

"What does your diet look like?" the doctor asked.

"Nothing too bad. I usually eat healthy stuff: smoothies, quinoa, salad . . ." I rattled off a list of things I could recall eating recently.

"Do you keep a food journal or track your eating habits?"

"No, I don't document anything, but I do make an effort to eat healthy!"

"Well, how much do you think you eat in a day?" the doctor asked.

"I don't know. Not very much. I'd guess around 1,200 to 1,500 calories. I don't eat a lot. I've been trying to lose weight," I confessed.

I could tell she wasn't convinced. "I see. Well, it might be a good idea to keep a food journal."

I left feeling puzzled, defeated, and, quite frankly, upset. The mere idea of a food journal irked me. *What a waste of time*, I thought. *Why do I need to document what I'm eating—doesn't she believe me? I am so sick of people assuming that if I just ate less, I'd be skinny. I'm barely eating anything!*

I didn't start journaling right away. I waited until I wasn't feeling as defensive and had warmed up to the idea just to prove I was right. I carried around a handy notebook throughout the day and meticulously documented each bite. My health-conscious breakfast at home, my fancy coffee during my hour-long commute, the bagels waiting in the breakroom, the daily lunch out with coworkers to escape the office, the afternoon snacks at my desk, the health-conscious dinner at home, the postworkday "glass" of wine. Turns out I was eating and drinking more than I thought I was. *A lot more.*

The food journal wasn't about convincing my doctor—it was about convincing myself. Day to day, I was eating well more than what my body could burn. My diet was far from perfect.

If you haven't already, I highly recommend starting a food log or journal to see what a typical day of eating looks like on paper. This is a great way to take immediate action.

Exploring Energy: Calories In, Calories Out

A calorie is a unit of energy used to describe nutritional requirement or consumption. You may have heard the phrase "calories in, calories out" in conversations about effective weight loss. And by now you may have realized that the world of fat loss, body composition, health, and nutrition is not as simplistic as "calories in, calories out." But that doesn't mean we can ignore the concept of energy balance altogether! Our overall calorie intake and individual energy expenditure determine whether we are balancing our needs, taking in excess, or falling short. Ultimately, this energy balance, surplus, or deficit is what drives our body weight.

Over time, an individual with a positive energy balance will store excess energy as triacylglycerols in adipose tissue, regardless of dietary macronutrient composition.[1] High carb, low carb, ketogenic, or otherwise, if you are taking in more energy than your body needs, it will be stored as body fat, and weight gain will ensue.

The same can be said for the opposite direction: Taking in less than your body needs will result in weight loss over time regardless of what you're actually eating. That's why the nutrition professor from Kansas State University who ate a calorie-reduced diet consisting of nothing but Twinkies, chips, and sugary snacks was able to lose 27 pounds (12.25 kg) in two months.[2] Was he advocating a snack-centric diet? No, clearly he had an ax to grind and a point to prove—that calories matter more than the nutritional value when it comes to *weight loss*. Am I recommending you drop this book and stock up on a lifetime supply of Twinkies

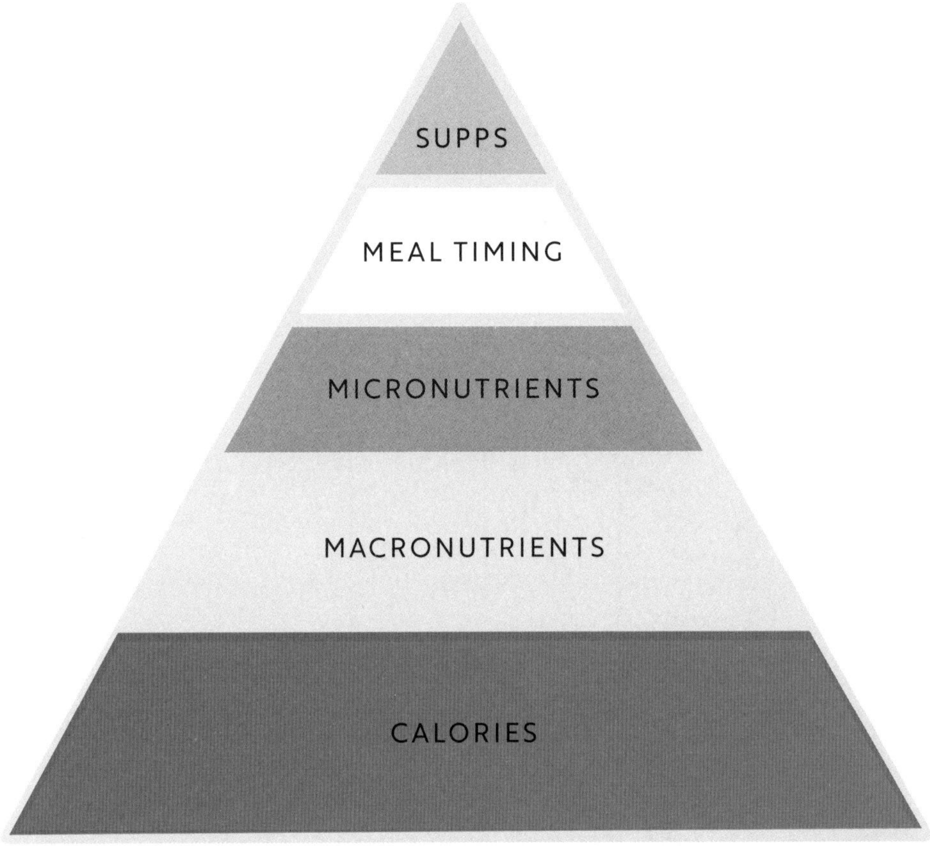
SUPPS
MEAL TIMING
MICRONUTRIENTS
MACRONUTRIENTS
CALORIES

EXCESS INTAKE IS STORED AS FAT	
Cause of Calorie Surplus	**Effect of Calorie Surplus**
Excess Dietary Fat	↑ body fat: excess fat directly stored ↑ fat-burning from diet ↓ fat-burning from adipose
Excess Carbohydrate	↑ body fat: dietary fat eaten with carbs is stored ↑ carb-burning from diet ↓ fat-burning from diet and adipose
Excess Protein	↑ body fat: dietary fat eaten with protein is stored ↑ protein-burning from diet ↓ fat-burning from diet and adipose
Excess Carbohydrate with Little Dietary Fat Intake	↑ body fat: carbs turn to fat for storage (de novo lipogenesis) ↑ carb-burning from diet ↓ fat-burning from adipose

Regardless of the macronutrient driving excess, energy intake beyond your needs is stored as body fat, as detailed in this chart.

instead? Not at all. I'm just reminding you that when it comes to gaining and losing weight, calories count.

Are calories the only thing that matters? Of course not. But completely disregarding their contribution isn't going to do us any good, either. The overall amount of food we eat on a keto diet absolutely affects our ability to lose weight. The concept of calories is often dismissed by the low-carb community, even viewed as taboo. There are undoubtedly more pieces to the puzzle than calories alone, but that doesn't mean energy balance should be discredited altogether. It should be considered an underlying principle of weight loss, maintenance, and gaining. After all, calories in, calories out just represents the fundamental thermodynamics of how our bodies exchange energy. Being aware of this basic energy exchange can help set you up for success and realistic expectations.

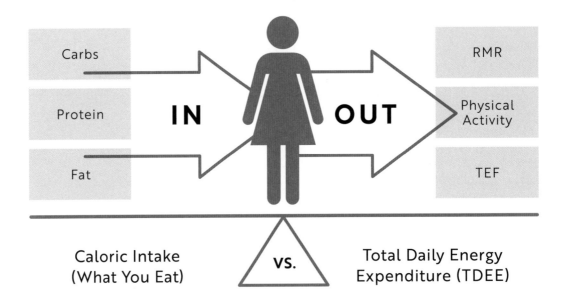

Carbs	RMR
Protein	Physical Activity
Fat	TEF

IN · **OUT**

Caloric Intake (What You Eat) · **VS.** · Total Daily Energy Expenditure (TDEE)

Calories In: Macronutrients

We already started to cover the *calories in* part of the equation at length in chapter 2. Remember: Macronutrients *are* the calories. With ketogenic diets, we are simply partitioning calorie intake in a way that supports efficient fat-burning. While the body becomes expert at utilizing fat for energy, the metabolic state of ketosis does not result in significant fat loss without a calorie deficit.

Calories Out: Metabolism and Physical Activity

While *calories in* represents our food intake, *calories out* is much more complex. We have more control over the amount of fuel we put into our bodies than we do over the fuel demands of our bodies. *Calories out* represents the overall amount of energy your body burns throughout the day. Total expenditure includes the energy required to fuel basic biological processes, support physical activity, and digest what you have eaten.

<u>Metabolic Rates for Women</u>

Your body is burning calories even when you aren't consciously doing anything. When you're lying completely still, dreaming about being best friends with Beyoncé (. . . just me?), your body is still using fuel to perform the rudimentary processes that keep you alive—such as breathing and making sure your heart doesn't stop beating. This basic energy demand is known as the basal metabolic rate (BMR), which accounts for the energy requirements to sustain organ function, respiration, blood circulation, and a wide variety of other basic life-sustaining processes. Your BMR accounts for the majority of your body's energy demands, making it the most significant contribution to your daily energy expenditure.

Basal metabolic rates can be determined under tightly controlled laboratory conditions, but that's not cost effective, practical, or even necessary. Resting metabolic rate (RMR) can be used to predict energy expenditure at rest based on weight, height, age, and sex using simple math formulas that are reasonably accurate. You will see that BMR and RMR are often used interchangeably.

Factors that affect metabolic rate include body composition, surface area, age, and gender. As women, this last point is of particular interest to us. Female bodies have lower metabolic rates than male bodies. This means our overall calorie needs are lower; if we expend less energy, we need to take in less energy—smaller portions, mindful measurements, lower-calorie options.

Though tragically unfair, the reason behind this is fairly straightforward. It primarily boils down to lean body mass. Lean body mass has higher metabolic activity than adipose tissue; those with more muscle and skeletal tissue burn more calories.[3] If you recall from the previous chapter, women have double the body fat of men. When all is equal—height, weight, and age—a man has greater lean body mass than a woman and, in turn, burns more calories at rest and during physical activity. This explains why men tend to lose weight faster than women, even with similar calorie deficits.[4] Comparing your weight loss progress and results to men's is futile. Don't!

If we go back to the car analogy from chapter 2, lean body mass is like a gas hog—it is the military-grade H1 Hummer that gets 9 miles per gallon in the city. The more of these gas hogs you own, the more you spend on fuel. Adipose tissue, on the other hand, is more like a Prius—it doesn't take as much fuel to sustain it.

As the primary determinant of metabolic rates and overall energy expenditure, preserving lean body mass should be at the forefront of our weight loss efforts. As women, we are already at a disadvantage when it comes to lean body mass; surely we want to do what we can to save our precious metabolically active tissue. Luckily, with adequate dietary protein intake, ketogenic diets have a protein-sparing effect that allows us to lose body fat while preserving lean mass, thus maintaining higher metabolic rates.[5]

Though gaining lean body mass is often a difficult feat, it is an effective way to raise your metabolism. Resistance training can be beneficial for increasing or maintaining lean body mass for women.[6] As we age, lean body mass declines and our metabolic rate dips further. Both endurance and strength training can be an effective way to combat the loss of lean tissue, even as we get older.[7] Staying physically active is imperative to preserving lean tissue, regardless of age.

Get Up and Move!
Depending on how active a person is, physical activity accounts for between 15 and 30 percent of total energy expenditure.[8] This includes both exercise and nonexercise activities involved in day-to-day living. Individual metabolic rate and intensity of the movements affect the amount of energy used to fuel these actions, but, as a rule, those who move more burn more calories.[9]

Examples of Exercise Activities	Examples of Nonexercise Activities
Dancing	Fidgeting
Running	Gardening
Swimming	Cleaning
Weight lifting	Standing
Cycling	Walking

In terms of calorie burn, the benefits of exercise and physical activity are clear. You don't have to run marathons or start powerlifting to benefit, either. If you're able, take the stairs instead of the elevator, stand at your desk instead of sitting all day, or choose the parking spot that's a little further away. Small, gradual changes can have a big impact over time.

Thermic Effect of Food: Protein Is King

The smallest contribution to energy expenditure involves the body's response to food. Though we are taking in energy while eating, we need energy input to process our food. Increased energy expenditure resulting from macronutrient metabolism is known as the thermic effect of food (TEF).

Each macronutrient has a different thermic effect on energy: Protein has the most significant impact, carbohydrates intermediate, and fat the least. In an average diet of mixed macronutrients, total energy expenditure is raised by approximately 10 percent due to TEF.[10] While TEF is a relatively small contribution to daily calorie needs, a practical takeaway here is that consumption of a high-protein meal burns more calories than a high-carb or high-fat meal.[11] Yet another reason not to shy away from protein.

Total Daily Energy Expenditure

Once you combine the calories burned from your basal or resting metabolic rate, your physical activity, and the thermic effect of food, you have the big-picture estimate of *calories out*. This sum is known as total daily energy expenditure (TDEE). Possible ways to increase this number include changing your body composition (i.e., gaining lean mass), becoming more physically active, and eating higher-protein meals. Just remember: No matter what you do to raise your energy needs, your food intake is going to determine whether you see the results you want.

Changes in your diet will provide the biggest bang for your buck. That's why you'll hear people say things like "Abs are made in the kitchen, not the gym" or "You can't out-train a bad diet." You can—and should!—engage in all sorts of things to keep your metabolism running at peak conditions, but if you aren't tackling the *calories in* portion, your results will disappoint you.

Total energy expenditure is the number that will form the basis of your macronutrient goals and calorie intake. Eating in balance with your TDEE will allow you to maintain your weight.

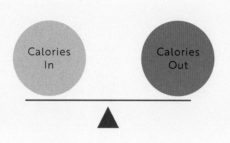

WEIGHT MAINTAINED

Isocaloric Balance
Energy In = Energy Out

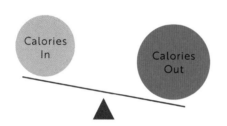

WEIGHT LOSS

Negative Caloric Balance
Energy In < Energy Out

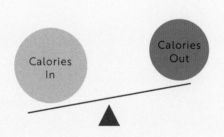

WEIGHT GAIN

Positive Caloric Balance
Energy In > Energy Out

THERMIC EFFECT OF FOOD (TEF)[12]	
Protein	20 to 30 percent
Carbs	5 to 10 percent
Fat	0 to 5 percent

Consuming over your TDEE will result in weight gain, while eating below your TDEE will create a calorie deficit that will enable you to lose weight. But beware: For reasons we will get into shortly, not all calorie deficits are created equal.

Dropping Calories Too Low

After all the fuss I've made about calories, you might assume that dramatically slashing your intake will bring the best results. But dropping calories too low can be problematic, especially for women. The more body fat you have, the safer it is for you to lower calories without losing lean body mass.

Very high calorie deficits can cause unnecessary stress on the body, which can make your hormones rage out, exacerbate any imbalances, and wreak havoc on your menstrual cycle. When this happens, it can feel like the body is fighting back against the calorie restriction. It is! A modest deficit is more appropriate and sustainable in most situations.

Is a Calorie Deficit Always Appropriate?

We talked about the reasons that cutting back on energy intake can be beneficial, but are there ever times when lowering your calorie intake is a bad idea? Yes!

Find Out Your Energy Expenditure

Curious what your TDEE is or how much energy is spent on certain activities? There are many easily accessible calculators online that can predict how many calories you burn based off your input. One is www.nal.usda.gov/fnic/calculators-and-counters.

If you're already at your ideal body weight and have chosen keto for reasons outside weight loss, there is no need for a calorie deficit.

Interested in strategically gaining weight to increase lean body mass? You will need a calorie surplus, not a deficit.

If you are exceptionally lean and don't have much body fat to lose, a calorie deficit may not be in your best interests, either. At some point, your energy requirements will be sapped from your lean tissue if the shortage persists. Once you reach your ideal body composition or become very lean, it's time to increase your calories to maintenance. You don't need to be on a perpetual calorie-restricted diet to maintain your progress; you just need to eat for your new body's needs.

HOW LOW CAN YOU GO?				
			Examples	
Calorie Deficit	Intensity	Safety	TDEE of 1,500	TDEE of 2,500
15 to 20 percent	Conservative	Safe	225 to 300 deficit 1,200 to 1,275 total intake	375 to 500 deficit 2,000 to 2,125 total intake
20 to 25 percent	Moderate	Low Risk	300 to 375 deficit 1,125 to 1,200 total intake	500 to 625 deficit 1,875 to 2,000 total intake
25 to 30 percent	Aggressive	Iffy	375 to 450 deficit 1,050 to 1,125 total intake	625 to 750 deficit 1,750 to 1,875 total intake
30+ percent	Extreme	Risky	450 to 1500 deficit up to 1,050 total intake	750 to 2,500 deficit up to 1,750 total intake

Here's how a daily calorie deficit may appear at different levels of restriction and energy expenditure. A short, sedentary woman may require much less energy than a woman who is taller, more muscular, or physically active. As you can see, your intake might look quite different from the next person. It all depends on your body.

Along the same lines, if you are a female athlete, it may be wise to forgo calorie restriction. Your body needs fuel. Undereating and overtraining is a recipe for disaster; often this combination leads to a medical condition known as the "female athlete triad," characterized by amenorrhea (loss of menstrual periods), osteoporosis, and disordered eating.[13] You don't need to be a competitive athlete for this to apply to you, either. Perhaps you enjoy endurance sports or tend to take exercise to the next level—without proper nutrition to fuel your physical activities, a calorie deficit puts you at risk.[14]

If you have an unresolved eating disorder, you don't need calorie restriction—full stop. You don't need to worry about calories; you need to work on your relationship with food. Putting any restriction on your diet won't benefit the real issue. Consider this your intervention, and please seek professional help. You're worth it.

What if you are pregnant? First of all, I do not recommend dieting during this period of your life. If you're pregnant and thinking about starting keto, reconsider drastic changes to your diet until after your bundle of joy has fully developed. You have different requirements, your food preferences fluctuate, and your hormones and body are already hard at work creating life. If you've become pregnant while eating a ketogenic diet and want to continue, that's ultimately between you and your doctor. There is little evidence showing whether ketogenic diets are suitable for pregnancy, as long-term effects and safety risks have yet to be established.[15] You want to make nutritious food choices, but your energy expenditure ramps up quite a bit during pregnancy and lactation.[16] Pregnancy is not the time to cut calories; you usually need to eat more, not less. Be patient—and congratulations, Mama!

Are you experiencing nutrient deficiencies? If you are having a hard time meeting nutritional needs, limited intake may prevent you from getting adequate vitamins, minerals, appropriate fatty acids, and amino acids. This can be avoided by carefully planning for nutritionally dense foods, but you might need to bump up your calories to give yourself room for more variety in addition to supplementation.

Lastly, if you find the transition to low-carb eating is difficult with a calorie deficit, hold off restricting your intake until your body has fully adapted to burning fat for fuel. The last thing you want to do is set yourself up for failure by taking on too many things at once. If keto and reduced calories are too much, hold off until you're ready.

The Devil Is in the Details: Common Calorie Mistakes

Before you start focusing on calories, let's take a minute to talk about two factors that trip people up: tracking calories and focusing too much on weight loss.

Macronutrients and Calorie Confusion: The 4/4/9 Rule
Once you begin paying attention to macronutrients, you will find accounting for their intake in grams will be the most efficient, accessible way to track them. First of all, macronutrient quantities appear as grams on nutrition labels and in nutrition databases. There are no conversions, ratios, or tricky math formulas involved—just simple addition that can be made even easier with mobile apps or nutrition software. More importantly, by dealing in grams, you concurrently count your calorie intake without running a completely separate tally.

But dealing with grams does run the potential to cause calorie confusion. To an untrained eye, a nutrition label with 10 grams of protein and 10 grams of fat appears to provide the same amount of calories per nutrient. This can be deceptive, as gram to gram, not all macronutrients offer the same number of calories.

Track with Technology

Mobile and desktop applications can be excellent resources for tracking nutrient intake. There are many to choose from, but I highly recommend Cronometer. This app tracks all things related to energy balance—calories, macronutrients, exercise—and other nutritionally important factors such as vitamins, minerals, fiber, amino acids, and fatty acids. And it's free! cronometer.com

Remember the 4/4/9 rule:

> Carbs have 4 calories per gram.
> Protein has 4 calories per gram.
> Fat has 9 calories per gram.

One gram of fat has more than twice as many calories as 1 gram of carbs or protein! In example on the previous page, the protein would have supplied 40 calories (4 calories × 10 grams) while the fat provided 90 calories (9 calories × 10 grams). Imagine the difference this makes in higher quantities! Racking up the fat grams can quickly add hundreds of calories to your daily intake, especially if you are mindlessly dousing your food with butter and oils in the name of keto.

Let's pretend someone is eating 120 grams of protein and 60 grams of fat while restricting their carb intake. Whoa—double the protein?! It might look like it in grams, but let's check the math to be sure we know where most of the energy comes from.

> **Protein:** 120 grams × 4 calories = 480 calories

> **Fat:** 60 grams × 9 calories = 540 calories

Even though it seems like protein is double the fat, based on grams, in this scenario, fat is still the primary source of dietary energy. If your head is spinning from all the math, don't worry. You won't have to tirelessly multiply each macronutrient gram you eat. That would be exhausting. I just want you to be aware of the 4/4/9 rule so when it comes to nutrition databases, labels, or apps, you can provide context to the numbers and choose accordingly.

We know calories matter, and it is very easy to slip into excess territory with calorie-dense fats. You will be eating plenty of fat on a ketogenic diet, but underestimating how many calories an ingredient contains is easy to do. Olive oil could effortlessly take you from a tablespoon serving size of 119 calories to several hundred calories with a heavy-handed pour.[17] Please note I'm not suggesting you avoid fat, just that you appropriately scale intake to avoid unintentional excess. On keto, fat is our primary source of energy, but it's still packed with calories. Mindfully tracking and measuring will help you lose body fat and meet your body composition goals by aligning how much you think you eat with how much you actually eat.

Focusing on Weight Loss

The 3,500-Calorie Misconception

If you are familiar with the concept of calories, then chances are high you have heard the conventional idea that one pound (454 g) equals 3,500 calories. One pound of what, exactly? This concept only holds true for body fat. The metabolizable energy found in 1 pound of stored carbohydrates or protein

Measure Your Portions

Measuring spoons, measuring cups, and kitchen scales aren't just for baking. To get a realistic sense of a portion or serving size, measure it. You might be surprised by the amounts.

Energy Scale for Food

Calories = Energy

CARBOHYDRATES:
4 Calories per gram

PROTEIN:
4 Calories per gram

FATS:
9 Calories per gram

HOW MANY CALORIES ARE THERE PER POUND?[20]	
Weight Component	Calories/Pound
Water	0
Glycogen	~1800
Muscle	600 to 700
Fat	3,500

in muscle is much lower than the same amount of fat, while a pound of water has no caloric value whatsoever.[18] The 3,500-calorie concept is a convenient estimate, but it doesn't represent the dynamic way we lose weight and is misrepresentative of actual weight loss.[19]

Weight Loss versus Fat Loss

Fat is more calorically dense than protein and carbs in food, and the same can be said for the energy in our body. In other words, it takes more energy to burn 1 gram of body fat than it does 1 gram of protein or carbs in our body (think: muscle or glycogen). What does this say about weight loss? It means it's a lot easier to lose muscle than body fat.

Your lean body mass, the calorie-burning furnace that determines your metabolic rate, can contribute to weight loss faster than the fat you're actually trying to get rid of. Gaining lean body mass is hard to do—just ask any bodybuilder. Losing lean mass, on the other hand, is quite easy if you're not careful about how you cut your calories.

A calorie deficit will cause weight loss, but what does that mean exactly? Weight loss is a combination of water, muscle, and fat. Without taking proper precautions, the number on the scale could be dropping without actually losing any body fat.

The number on the scale only reflects the Earth's gravitational pull relative to your body. It has little to do with what your body is actually made of. The number is continuously fluctuating—particularly for women!—depending on the time of day, where you are in your menstrual cycle, or what you've recently eaten. As someone who has been overweight, underweight, and everywhere in between, I'd also argue this number is the least interesting thing about you.

My advice: Quit focusing on weight loss. Weight loss can be achieved through wacky ways of cutting calories, starving yourself, and other unhealthy approaches. If you want to see dramatic improvements in your body composition, fat loss reigns supreme.

Glycogen Depletion (a.k.a. "Water Weight")

When you first start keto, your body will burn through your glycogen stores over the first few days. This depletion of stored carbohydrates will result in decreased weight from losses

A Tale of Two Keto Dieters

Once there were identical twin sisters, Julie and Kate. Taking their twinning to new heights, the sisters start keto at the same time. Their weight has been steadily decreasing in a parallel fashion.

Julie reads about something called "fat fasting," a ketogenic crash diet, and decides to try it. While she does, Kate continues eating her moderate calorie deficit paired with adequate protein, carbs from fibrous veggies, and fat for satiety.

At the end of the week, Julie calls Kate. "Kate, you'll never believe it. Fat really does make you skinny. I lost 5 pounds (2.27 kg) this week!"

"Tell me everything!" Kate is excited to learn her twin's new diet trick, especially after she was so diligent and only lost 1 pound (454 g).

"Basically, I just drank butter all week long," Julie replies.

The two laugh maniacally—the way sisters do—and vow to repeat the butter-drinking experiment.

But what really happened here?

Kate kept her calorie deficit around 500 calories per day. She went to the gym, ate sufficient protein and nutrient-dense veggies, and measured her portions. She did everything right, so what gives?

Kate lost 1 pound (454 g) of body fat. She should be celebrating.

> 500-calorie deficit per day × 7 days = 3,500-calorie deficit for the week
>
> 1 pound (45 g) of body fat = 3,500 calories
>
> 3,500-calorie deficit ÷ 3,500 calories per pound of fat = 1 pound fat loss

Meanwhile, Julie drank butter all week. Her calorie intake worked out to a daily deficit of 500 calories, too, but she didn't have time for the gym. Without adequate dietary protein, Julie's body was unable to source amino acids from her diet, so her body turned to muscle to satisfy its basic protein requirements. As each day passed, she lost more muscle tissue. While a pound of fat provides 3,500 calories in energy, a pound of muscle ranges from 600 to 700 calories. Let's check the math again.

> 500-calorie deficit per day × 7 days = 3,500-calorie deficit for the week
>
> 1 pound (454 g) of muscle = 700 calories
>
> 3,500-calorie deficit ÷ 700 calories per pound of muscle = 5-pound (2.3 kg) muscle loss

Kate clearly came out on top in this situation, regardless of total weight loss.

Of course, Kate and Julie aren't real people and their story has been dramatized, but this scenario plays out regularly in the low-carb and ketogenic communities. Advice to eat more fat for quicker weight loss or fat fasting to break a weight loss stall runs rampant. This way of thinking is backward. Sure, you might be able to lose more weight, but at what expense? You are left with less lean body mass than you started with. Your metabolic rate is slower. You burn even fewer calories than you did before. When people say that dieting "destroys your metabolism," this is exactly what they mean.

of both glycogen and water. Per each gram of glycogen stored, there are at least 3 grams of water that accompany it.[21] Your body will also release large amounts of water as sodium retention drops during carb restriction (see chapter 12).

Let's say you burn through 1 pound (454 g) of glycogen, and you have three times as much water that's released as well—that's 4 pounds (1.8 kg) of weight that has nothing to do with body fat in addition to the extra water expelled with sodium. This is one primary reason people see such rapid weight loss on low-carb diets in the beginning stages.[22] It's also why people seem to immediately "gain it all back" once they start eating carbohydrates again—as the glycogen stores refill and sodium is retained, water comes along as well. This is not fat loss or gain; this is merely one way your weight will fluctuate when eating a ketogenic diet and yet another example of why you shouldn't rely on your scale to paint the full picture.

Instead of measuring your progress by weight, a much safer and more effective way to gauge improvements is to measure changes in your body composition. How much lean mass are you working to save, and how much fat can you spare to lose? This will help bring focus to healthy changes in your body composition and realistic goal setting.

You don't want to set a goal weight of 120 pounds (54.5 kg) if you have 120 pounds of lean body mass, right? Not only would 0 percent body fat be detrimental to your health, but it's also not really in the realm of attainable body goals. Place your focus on fat loss and the results you truly desire will rise to the forefront.

Measuring at Home
You can get body fat testing done at home or at your gym using calipers, which measure skin folds at specific sites to estimate body composition. They can be tricky to use, and some areas of the body naturally hold more fat, which can affect accuracy.

BODY COMPOSITION IN WOMEN	
Essential fat	10 to 14 percent
Top athlete	15 to 20 percent
In shape	21 to 24 percent
Healthy	25 to 32 percent
Overweight	33 percent and higher

Bioelectrical impedance is another approach that can be done at home. Devices that measure this send an electrical current through the body to gauge body composition; lean mass conducts the electrical impulses, while fat mass impedes the flow of electricity. Low-cost handheld devices are available, and some scales have this as a built-in feature. Hydration and electrolyte balance are key factors to an accurate reading.

Another home option is the circumference method. This involves measuring the circumference of key areas and using a formula to predict your body composition. A reliable tool for women to use is the U.S. Navy body composition formula.[23] Measurements are taken at the neck, natural waist, and hips on bare skin—all you need is a flexible tape measure and a couple of minutes to plug in your data. Use an online calculator to make quick work of the calculations, such as the one found at www.calculator.net/body-fat-calculator.html.

Measuring at a Facility

If you want the most accurate measurements, try a testing facility. The downside is that these tests can be expensive and challenging to find in some locations.

If you are going to splurge on testing, dual-energy X-ray absorption (DEXA) scans are the gold standard.[24] In addition to body fat and lean mass measurements for your whole body, DEXA scans provide detailed information about bone density. This can give insight into your bone health and risk for osteopenia and osteoporosis.

5

The Female Hormonal Cycle

We can't properly discuss keto, women's health, nutrition, or fat loss without talking about hormones. But what exactly are they? Hormones are the chemical messengers responsible for orchestrating many processes in our bodies. When they're balanced, your hormone levels are healthy and able to provide optimal support for bodily functions. The body thrives in this state. A hormonal imbalance occurs when there is too much, or too little, of a particular hormone.

The systems in the body are all intimately interconnected, and an imbalance in just one thing can have a ripple effect, causing multiple processes to go awry. In many cases, even small hormonal problems can have serious repercussions. If one part of the system is broken, the impact can be widespread. When chemical messages aren't adequately relayed, many of the mechanisms that ensure our body runs correctly risk dysfunction.

As women, our hormones fluctuate cyclically throughout the month by nature; there is an ebb and flow of estrogen and progesterone. This keeps our reproductive health in tip-top shape while interweaving with many other biologically important processes, including some that affect our ability to store or lose body fat.

Diet and lifestyle can affect our hormones, which is excellent news once we know how to optimize this for our benefit. Eating a ketogenic diet can dramatically affect our hormones, so we need to do our part to ensure it is a positive shift and not one that throws us into hormonal chaos. Considering how a woman's body responds to a ketogenic diet, calorie restriction, and the oscillations brought on by each hormonal cycle allows us to implement the diet in a way that promotes the balance required to flourish. The goal is not to reach an ideal body composition at all costs but to lose excess body fat safely, without sacrificing hormonal health. A better body *and* happy hormones—you can have both!

In chapter 6, we'll discuss even more of the key hormonal players that contribute to body composition and overall hormonal balance. But, for now, let's focus on one of the fundamental differences between male and female bodies: our sex hormones.

Male versus Female Sex Hormones

First, let me clarify a common misconception: everyone has both "male" and "female" sex hormones. Estrogens are associated with females and androgens with males; however, these hormones are both present in both men and women, just in varying degrees. Women predominantly produce estrogens and progesterone, the two female sex hormones. Some amount of the male hormone testosterone is also present in women, though it is created and needed in much smaller quantities. The reverse is true for men: Men have high testosterone levels, with minor estrogen and progesterone requirements.

Testosterone: The Male Sex Hormone
Testosterone levels in women are much lower than in men, though the hormone does play a critical role in our bodies. Testosterone is essential to our lean body mass, libido, and even blood cell production, but too much can spell trouble—acne, facial hair, hair loss, and fat deposition around the abdomen similar to what is seen in men.[1] High levels of testosterone can also interfere with our menstrual cycles and fertility.[2]

Testosterone levels are not subject to wild fluctuations during each cycle the way progesterone and estrogen are, but the hormone does peak before ovulation. The result is an increased libido during the most fertile time in our cycle, nature's way of trying to get us pregnant. Yet another remnant of our evolutionary survival strategy for reproductive success. Overall, women don't see a dramatic rise and fall in testosterone levels, so the hormone's impact on bodily processes remains fairly consistent. The ratio of the hormone in relation to the female sex hormones can be an important factor in hormonal balance.

Estrogen and Progesterone: The Yin and Yang
What do our primary sex hormones do? One of their main jobs is to prepare the uterus for menstruation or pregnancy. But in addition to their essential role in our menstrual

cycles, estrogen and progesterone are involved in regulation of appetite, body weight, energy expenditure, carbohydrate metabolism, and insulin sensitivity. These hormones are responsible for breast development and female fat distribution, where more fat is deposited in the hips and thighs.[3]

In many respects, estrogen and progesterone have seemingly opposing functions—the actions of estrogen are often countered by progesterone. However, the two hormones aren't rivaling forces in our bodies. They operate in a complementary fashion, each counterbalancing the other—progesterone acting as the yin to estrogen's yang. We need both. Progesterone often "turns off" estrogen after it has done its job, which is hugely important for the overall balance our bodies are trying to achieve. We'll look at how these two hormones fluctuate throughout each cycle and what that means for us shortly.

In women, these sex hormones are produced primarily in the ovaries, though other glands and tissues engage in their production. In addition to the ovaries, many tissues can synthesize estrogens, including adipose tissue, our stored body fat.[4] The majority of progesterone is also manufactured in the ovaries, though adrenal glands and other tissues participate in progesterone synthesis depending on life stages. During pregnancy, for example, progesterone is one of the most important hormones synthesized by the placenta.[5]

Because adipose tissue can contribute significantly to the estrogen pool, particularly after menopause, high body fat percentages and obesity promote elevated levels of estrogen.[6] This has been proven to be a critical factor in hormone imbalance and can put women at risk for chronic inflammation and breast cancer.[7] Maintaining healthy body fat levels is an essential element of restoring hormonal balance.

Reduce Body Fat for Hormonal Balance

When it comes to harmony among your hormones, reducing body fat is a vital piece to the puzzle if you are above a healthy body weight.

The Menstrual Cycle: Let's Talk About Periods!

What fun is a book for women if we don't get to discuss our periods? If you hate talking lady business, bear with me—this is important stuff.

Much like a vital sign—pulse, body temperature, blood pressure, or respiratory rate—our menstrual cycle offers regular feedback and clues about what's going on in our body. A normal menstrual cycle suggests balanced hormones, while irregularities and complications are indicative of a hormonal imbalance and underlying health issues.[8]

The Ideal Menstrual Cycle

Although menstrual cycles vary from woman to woman, the average is approximately 28 days in length. Our cycles can be divided into two phases that are separated by ovulation, when an ovary releases an egg into the fallopian tube.

Preovulation: The Follicular Phase (Days 1 to 14)

The preovulatory phase begins when you start your menstrual bleed, which typically lasts 3 to 7 days. During this time and up until ovulation, follicle-stimulating hormone (FSH) is released by the pituitary gland, the master endocrine gland of the body. The FSH stimulates the growth of ovarian follicle cells and prompts these cells to secrete estrogen into the bloodstream. The follicle cells continue to grow in this phase of the menstrual cycle, causing estrogen levels to surge. The first phase of your cycle is dominated by estrogen. As estrogen levels rise, your uterine lining begins to build gradually.

Ovulation occurs around day 14, when the pituitary stops secreting FSH and switches over to secretion of luteinizing hormone (LH). This hormonal switch signals the follicle cells to release the egg from the ovary. Once the egg pops out, you are in the second phase of the cycle and you can get pregnant if the egg is fertilized by the time it reaches your uterus—this is when you are most fertile.

Postovulation: The Luteal Phase (Days 14 to 28)

The postovulatory phase is the second half of the cycle, beginning once the follicle cells start receiving messages from LH instead of the FSH. LH tells the follicle cells (now called "corpus luteum") to start secreting progesterone. As a result, estrogen secretion sharply declines, while progesterone levels soar. Your core body temperature also increases.

Progesterone's primary job in the menstrual cycle is to grow the endometrial blood vessels in preparation for pregnancy, lining the uterus with lush, dense vascularization waiting to receive an embryo. If an egg is fertilized, it can implant into this nourishing landscape for further development. If it isn't, the previously grown follicle cells shrink, secreting less and less progesterone as the cells deteriorate. Around day 28, the corpus luteum follicle cells have shriveled up and stopped secreting progesterone altogether, causing the lining to shed and menstrual bleed to commence. Now we're back to square one, at the beginning of the ovulatory phase, and the cycle repeats.

Tracking Your Period

This whole cycle is designed to prepare our bodies for pregnancy. Remember, biologically, we are geared toward optimal reproductive success. Regular periods signal health and vitality.

Tracking your cycle throughout the month is a great way to get in tune with your body and assess your hormonal health. The simplest way to do this is with an app on your phone or computer. There are a variety of free options that help you track your cycle, energy levels, and mood. They can even predict your next period.

Due to the bleeding, your period is a reasonably easy thing to track by sight alone. The time from day one bleed to day one bleed equals your cycle length. However, the different stages of your cycle may not be as obvious—they aren't always split directly in half. To key

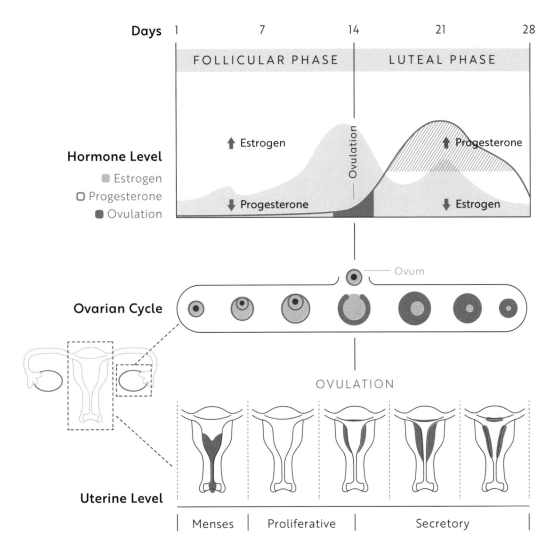

Days 1   7   14   21   28

FOLLICULAR PHASE   LUTEAL PHASE

Hormone Level
⬤ Estrogen
◻ Progesterone
⬤ Ovulation

⬆ Estrogen   Ovulation   ⬆ Progesterone

⬇ Progesterone   ⬇ Estrogen

Ovum

Ovarian Cycle

OVULATION

Uterine Level

| Menses | Proliferative | Secretory |

in on when you ovulate and transition into the second phase of your cycle, monitor your temperature daily. A reading of 99.6° F (38° C) after steadily measuring 98.6° F (37° C) can alert you to the change—it's like the basal body temperature method of birth control. You could also use a home test kit for the luteinizing hormone (LH) to track ovulation, which is more accurate than relying on temperature alone.

The Menstrual Cycle and Your Diet

Besides clueing you in to overall health, is your menstrual cycle essential to pay attention to for any other reason? One hundred percent yes! Hormonal fluctuations related to your cycle play a significant role in your metabolism, insulin sensitivity, and food preferences—and, in turn, your ability to lose and store body fat.

Menstruation and Metabolic Rate

Your metabolic rate, the necessary number of calories required to sustain your body, is lower in the first phase of your cycle than the second phase. During the preovulatory, or follicular, phase of your menstrual cycle, your basal metabolic rate (BMR) drops. The drop in metabolism occurs during the menstrual bleed but is most significant in the week before ovulation.[9] The metabolic rate then gradually rises, increasing during the second half of your menstrual cycle.[10]

The rise in metabolism during the postovulatory phase is related to progesterone levels, which increase both body temperature and energy expenditure as new tissue is grown in the endometrial lining.[11] Knowing this fundamental shift in metabolic rate can help you understand how you might adjust your own "calories in, calories out" equation.

Fewer calories are burned at rest during the first phase of your cycle, while more calories are burned in the second phase, after ovulation. You can use this information to adjust your activity levels and food intake accordingly.

Change in Eating Habits During Menstrual Cycle

Food intake is influenced by a wide variety of factors, including hormones, so it's no surprise our menstrual cycles affect what and how much we eat. Though the mechanisms are still being explored, several studies have shown appetite and energy intake in women are closely tied to their cycles.[12]

For one, there is a significant increase in caloric intake during the luteal phase of the menstrual cycle.[13] This makes sense given the fact that our metabolic rate rises during this time—your body senses it needs more fuel and signals you to eat more. However, the increased calorie burn during the second phase of your cycle will be canceled out if you aren't mindful of your calorie intake. Regularly allowing your appetite to overcompensate for the extra calories your body is using up can lead to increased body fat over time.

The lower calorie intake of the first half of the cycle offset by higher consumption in the second half also suggests that estrogen and progesterone play a role in appetite regulation. When estrogen levels are high, appetite is suppressed; as progesterone rises, the appetite is stimulated.[14]

This is also the time when intense food cravings rear their ugly head. Chocolate, sweet, salty, fatty—studies have repeatedly shown that food cravings skyrocket during the luteal phase.[15] If you've ever found yourself at the bottom of a freshly opened ice cream container before your period, this could explain why.

Estrogen levels are linked to serotonin and dopamine, the feel-good chemicals in our body related to happiness, well-being, and reward.[16] As estrogen levels take a dive in the second phase of the menstrual cycle, so does our mood! Food cravings are symptoms of a reward-driven appetite to increase serotonin and dopamine—this is our body's attempt to make us feel better.[17] Progesterone is also linked to these neurotransmitters.[18] This gives us insight into the rise of premenstrual syndrome, or PMS, building up to the days before your period and the amplification of food cravings as estrogen and progesterone levels both plummet before the next cycle begins.

Ketogenic diets can have an appetite-suppressing effect, which is particularly helpful when appetite and food cravings grow stronger in the second phase of the cycle.

Food Metabolism and Insulin Sensitivity
The menstrual cycle also affects our sensitivity to the insulin hormone and, in turn, our insulin resistance. In the beginning half of the cycle, we are more sensitive to the effects of insulin and therefore able to take up glucose into the cells more effectively. This means that in the follicular phase, before ovulation, women are better able to efficiently metabolize carbohydrates for energy.[19] One reason for this is that estrogen increases insulin sensitivity.[20] If you are going to eat carbohydrates, the ideal time to do so is in the first phase of your menstrual cycle.

As progesterone levels rise and estrogen dips in the second phase of the cycle, we lose this sensitivity and become more insulin resistant.[21] Insulin resistance impairs our ability to properly metabolize carbohydrates for energy, thereby increasing blood sugar, insulin levels, and fat storage during this time when a high-carbohydrate diet is consumed. Choosing low-carb foods is an effective way to bypass the impaired glucose uptake. As previously discussed, arguably one of the biggest benefits of a ketogenic diet is the alternative metabolic pathway to combat a faulty insulin response. Eating a keto diet during times of insulin resistance can help alleviate the effects of insulin resistance, balancing blood sugar and hormones.

The thermic effect of food (TEF) decreases in the second phase of the menstrual cycle as well, possibly as a result of inhibited glucose uptake and slower transit of food through the digestive tract.[22] If you recall from chapter 4, TEF is part of our "calories out" equation and protein scores the highest TEF of all the macronutrients. To counteract the decrease in TEF, we can choose higher-protein foods to increase the digestive impact on calorie burn.

Keto is very beneficial during your luteal phase. Eating fewer carbs with higher protein and fat can help combat the increased insulin resistance in the second half of your cycle to balance blood sugar and hormones.

Diet Starts . . . Tomorrow?
You can start keto whatever time suits you best, but consider starting your diet during the follicular phase of your cycle. After your menstrual bleed has ended and your estrogen is rising, you may have better compliance with your new dietary choices.

That's right: Impulsiveness can be affected by which part of the menstrual cycle you are in. Rising levels of estrogen in the follicular phase are related to decreased impulsive behavior compared to stages of the cycle when estrogen is low.[23] As estrogen levels fall in the second phase of the cycle, impulsive behavior rises. This time also coincides with increased food cravings, which can further provoke impulsive eating behavior.[24] Even with the best intentions, the combination of increased appetite, intense cravings, and impulsiveness can lead to excess intake and crush our efforts to even get started on a diet. Beginning your diet when estrogen levels are at their peak in the follicular phase of your cycle may help you battle the urge to quit your diet before you even get started.

Menstruation and Body Weight

This may not come as a surprise if you've ever struggled to zip up your jeans in the days leading up to your period, but fluid retention patterns are closely linked to the menstrual cycle as well. Water retention, or bloating, escalates near the end of the luteal phase. In the days leading up to the period bleed, fluid retention soars as the levels of progesterone and estrogen plummet, finally peaking on the first day of menstrual flow.[25] The amount of bloating wanes as the period continues and the excess water retained by the body is reduced. By mid–follicular phase, things will have returned to normal, and bloating is alleviated.[26]

As you may suspect, this extra retained fluid can affect your weight. Bear in mind, this water weight is just that—weight. It's not body fat, it's not muscle, it's only temporary fluid adding to

YOUR PERIOD'S EFFECTS		
Effect on:	During Follicular Phase (Pre-ovulation)	During Luteal Phase (Postovulation)
Dominant hormone	Estrogen	Progesterone
Metabolic rate	Lower	Higher
Calorie intake	Lower	Higher
Food cravings	Lower	Higher
Thermic effect of food (TEF)	Higher	Lower
Insulin sensitivity	Higher	Lower
Impulsiveness	Lower	Higher

This chart provides a brief snapshot of how the hormonal influences of your menstrual cycle impact your diet and metabolism.

the number on the scale. It will soon be gone and out of your life for good—or at least until next month. So, that said, here's another friendly reminder to stop paying so much attention to your weight.

<u>Keeping Your Body Image in Check</u>

Despite these completely *normal, natural* shifts in fluid retention during the menstrual cycle, studies have shown these changes negatively impact body image.[27] When studying the menstrual phase and body perceptions, researchers found reports of body dissatisfaction correlated with fluid retention leading up to and during the period.[28] Negative thoughts about the body, anxiety over appearance, and skewed perception of body size were observed even though there were *no significant changes* in actual body composition.[29]

Simply knowing your weight will fluctuate without a change in body fat can help you set realistic expectations for your body. But sometimes perception outweighs logic and body image takes a nosedive. It's good to have a self-love plan in place just in case you find yourself teetering into territory where you beat yourself up over something you have little control over. Try shifting the time and energy you spend criticizing yourself to healthy activities instead. Make a self-care list full of positive actions that center on you and make you feel wonderful. For example, write down something positive about yourself. Explore a nearby park or trail. Give yourself a manicure or treat yourself at the salon. Grab a book and plunge into a cozy bath. Write down positive affirmations and repeat them when you start to feel the negative energy creeping back. It can be anything that makes you feel good!

Menstrual Irregularities and Absence: You Don't Know What You've Got Till It's Gone

So, what if you don't fall into the cookie-cutter, textbook menstrual cycle previously outlined? Welcome to the club, sister. Millions of women of reproductive age experience menstrual dysfunction.

What if your menstrual cycle lasts only two weeks?
What if it's drawn out over two months?
What if you bleed longer than a week?
What if you don't bleed at all?

What's really to blame in these scenarios? You guessed it: a hormone imbalance. Wonky hormones are responsible for driving these symptoms, and, in most cases, estrogen is the culprit. Don't read this the wrong way; estrogen is a hugely important hormone for us, and we need it for all kinds of things: fertility, glucose metabolism, a healthy immune system, and cardiovascular health, just to name a few. But too much or too little estrogen can be problematic in many ways, and this estrogen imbalance is at the epicenter of nearly all human pathologies.[30]

Imbalanced estrogen, metabolic, autoimmune, degenerative, and even infectious levels are linked to many chronic diseases.[31] For premenopausal women, elevated estrogen is often the perpetrator. Luckily, ketogenic diets can help restore hormonal balance.[32]

Excess Estrogen: Too Much Yang

We live in an estrogen-saturated world. Estrogens and estrogen-like chemicals are in our food supply and throughout our environment. These additional estrogens all contribute to increased estrogen levels.[33] They work their way up the food chain and into our meals, and we are bathed in them throughout our environment; this compounds over time, and, as a result, our hormones are a mess.

And the estrogen-like compounds that aren't really estrogens? They have a chemical structure so similar to our own estrogen they are able to bind to the same receptors in our body and mimic the effects of actual estrogens. This leads to an overexpression of the hormone and fuels estrogen dominance.[34]

In women, high estrogen can potentially lead to polycystic ovarian syndrome (PCOS), endometriosis, obesity, breast cancer, and ovarian cancer.[35] Symptoms of high estrogen levels that are easily detected include weight gain, PMS, heavy periods, breast tenderness, and fibroids.[36]

In our food supply, estrogens can be found in both plant and animal products. Soy, for example, is a well-known plant-based source of estrogen. In traditional preparations, soy is often fermented, which dramatically improves the nutritional profile, but in our modern food supply, it often goes unfermented and is often highly processed. The components in soy can enhance or inhibit our natural estrogen,[37] which can be a double-edged sword when trying to conquer a hormonal imbalance. Phytoestrogens can help normalize hormone levels; when estrogen is high, they can out-compete the body's estrogen and lower the estrogenic action. In premenopausal women, soy and other phytoestrogens often act against estrogen. But during and after menopause, when estrogen is low, phytoestrogens act like estrogens and provide a natural boost.[38]

Of course, animal products also provide a source of estrogen. Animals raised on hormones can be a significant contributor to the incoming hormone load. In a study comparing hormone levels in beef, estrogen levels of U.S. beef were six-hundred times higher than those of Japanese beef![39] The explanation for this is simple: Ninety-seven percent of beef cattle in the United States receive steroid implants, an uncommon practice in Japan.[40] Though they certainly aren't in the majority, there are farmers throughout the United States who choose to raise their animals without the use of added steroid hormones. Due to consumer demand, even the big corporations are starting to offer hormone-free alternatives. You have options. By choosing animal products raised without hormone supplementation, you can further reduce your incoming estrogen burden.

In addition to choosing animal products raised without hormones, you may also want to consider limiting dairy intake. Steroid hormones, such as estrogen, can easily pass from the blood into milk. In fact, the primary sources of animal-derived estrogens in the diet are milk and dairy products, accounting for 60 to 70 percent.[41] If you do choose to include dairy in your diet, then selecting options from animals raised without hormones is your best bet.

There are also estrogen-like compounds in our environment that can increase the estrogen load. For example, Bisphenol A (BPA), found in plastics, can leach into water, causing estrogenic effects.[42] Plastic water bottles, food containers, canned foods and drinks, and even baby bottles can be sources of BPA exposure.[43] Pesticides, such as herbicides and insecticides, have also been found to be endocrine disruptors, increasing estrogenic effects and affecting hormonal balance.[44]

Lifestyle factors can also contribute to excess estrogen. I hate to be a buzzkill, but even moderate amounts of alcohol consumption can elevate estrogen levels.[45] If you are on a hormone-balancing mission, it's best to steer clear. While I'm on the subject, alcohol won't do you any favors in the fat loss department, either (see page 166).

Not only can obesity be a result of high levels of estrogen, but obesity in and of itself can swing estrogen levels into the red. Insulin resistance is also a contributing factor in unfavorable rises in estrogen. Insulin resistance and obesity decrease levels of the hormone that binds free estrogen and testosterone, the sex hormone binding globulin (SHBG). If SHBG isn't available to secure the sex hormones, you end up with an overabundance of free estrogen and testosterone. This leads to further hormone imbalance. Addressing insulin resistance and obesity can lower levels of estrogen and testosterone by increasing SHBG. Estrogen levels have been found to decrease proportionally with weight loss.[46]

Low Progesterone: Not Enough Yin

Too Much Estrogen

Excess estrogen levels provide feedback to the body to reduce FSH secretion, the follicle-stimulating hormone that signals the ovarian follicle cells to kick into gear and grow during the first phase of the menstrual cycle.[47] Limited FSH means follicle cell growth is also limited, which can significantly affect the menstrual cycle and hormones. If the follicle cells are unable to grow, this can lead to anovulation, where ovulation does not occur at all.[48]

As a result, the menstrual cycle doesn't progress into the second phase—no corpus luteum, no progesterone. If you aren't

How to Avoid Excess Estrogen

- Avoid eating or drinking dairy products, processed soy, and hormone-raised animal products.
- Use BPA-free containers.
- Choose organically grown produce.
- Reduce your alcohol intake.
- If you're dealing with obesity, lose weight—a ketogenic diet is a great way!

High levels of cortisol lead to low levels of progesterone, which is one reason you can lose your period if you are under a lot of stress or undereating.

ovulating, you aren't making progesterone. This is just one explanation for low progesterone levels, with effects that include infertility, missed periods, or no periods at all.

Signs of low progesterone include no luteal phase or a short luteal phase (which can be detected if you are tracking your periods), PMS, premenstrual bleeding, spotting, prolonged bleeding, or heavy periods. Low progesterone is also associated with polycystic ovarian syndrome (PCOS), fibroids, acne, hair loss, anxiety, depression, migraines, and perimenopause in women in their thirties and forties.[49] Without progesterone to balance the effects of estrogen, weight gain can also occur.

Estrogen excess can contribute to low progesterone, so the methods used to reduce estrogens may sometimes benefit progesterone levels.

Hormonal Birth Control

Hormonal birth control is another widespread cause of low progesterone in women of reproductive age. The synthetic hormones in birth control shut down our natural hormone production, suppressing FSH and LH production to prevent ovulation. No ovulation, no pregnancy—it's effective if you are trying not to get pregnant. But without FSH or LH, production of estrogen and progesterone is also prevented.

Hormonal birth control provides synthetic versions of estrogen, but some types also supply progestin, a man-made version of progesterone. It's essentially hormone replacement therapy, though most women taking birth control are plenty capable of producing their own hormones, and the synthetic versions aren't actually identical replacements. Progestins are similar to progesterone, but small variations in the chemical structure cause them to behave differently in the body—they don't deliver the same messages as natural progesterone. With hormonal birth control, you either don't get any progesterone at all or get a synthetic replacement that's not particularly helpful at balancing the effects of estrogen. However, many women find that hormonal birth control mitigates erratic patterns of wildly dysfunctional periods or helps to manage the symptoms of endometriosis. Consider your personal context and work with your healthcare provider to determine the best course of action.

While hormonal birth control is often the big bandage prescribed to "fix" your periods or hormonal imbalances, it isn't actually *fixing* anything. If anything, hormonal birth control further drives imbalances. The synthetic hormones simply treat the symptoms and do not address the root cause of the issue. A chemically induced cycle that creates the illusion of a normal functioning menstrual cycle is *not a normal functioning menstrual cycle*. The underlying problems are still there. Before you hop on birth control to regulate your periods, weigh the impact it will have on your natural hormone production and balance. Many forms of birth control aren't hormonally driven; consider a hormone-free alternative to prevent unwanted pregnancies. Copper IUDs, barrier methods, and fertility awareness are a few options. Discuss alternatives with your health care practitioner to determine what is right for you.

Stress

Stress can affect your menstrual cycle by way of the stress hormone cortisol, which we will talk about in more detail in the next chapter. When you think of stress, you might imagine overwhelming emotional pressure. But in addition to emotional stress, your body interprets all kinds of things as stressors—illness, a severe drop in calorie intake, lack of sleep, trauma, and so on. Your body releases cortisol as a way of handling these challenges; it's a survival mechanism as part of our fight-or-flight response. Cortisol competes with progesterone, meaning the hormones are in a tug-of-war with each other. High levels of cortisol lead to low levels of progesterone, which is one reason you can lose your period if you are under a lot of stress or undereating. That's another reason to avoid dropping calories too low.

Perimenopause

As you age, your progesterone levels slowly decline. You might suspect a steady decrease in estrogen levels to accompany this change, but that doesn't come until later on. In the years leading up to menopause, our progesterone levels tank while our estrogens remain high. As a result, our natural ability to counterbalance estrogen decreases. The ratio of estrogen to progesterone is skewed, and it's not in our favor.

Even with entirely normal levels of estrogen, this imbalance can lead to signs and symptoms of estrogen excess. To balance things out, many women choose to supplement with bioidentical progesterone. Unlike its synthetic friend (or foe), progestin, bioidentical progesterone is, as the name implies, biologically equivalent to our natural progesterone and has the same effects. If you are in your mid-thirties to -forties and have low progesterone, consider a progesterone supplement during your luteal phase. But beware of imitations. You want progesterone—not progestin, not progestogen—P-R-O-G-E-S-T-E-R-O-N-E. Talk to your health care provider to discuss whether progesterone supplementation is appropriate for you.

If you read the word "perimenopause" and your eyes glazed over because you aren't quite there yet or if you think menopause is light years away—HAHAHA. This natural drop in progesterone can begin as early as the mid-thirties. I encourage you to become familiar with how your hormones change with age. You won't be young forever (sad, I know); stay ahead of your hormonal fluctuations instead of letting them sneak up on you.

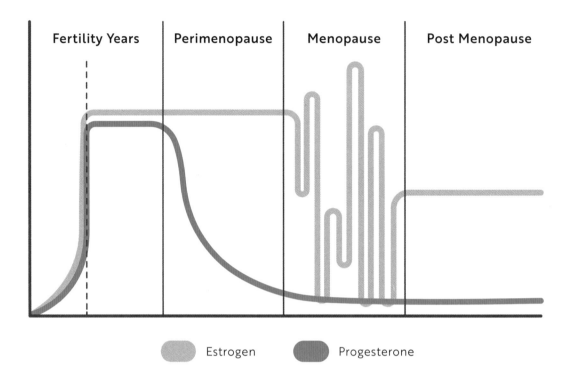

| Fertility Years | Perimenopause | Menopause | Post Menopause |

Estrogen   Progesterone

Menopause

With all its lovely side effects—hot flashes, weight gain, fatigue, night sweats, irritability, depression, osteoporosis, decreased sex drive, insomnia, vaginal dryness, hair loss, brain fog, anxiety—it's no wonder so many women don't talk about this particular phase of their life. Eighty-four percent of women surveyed by the AARP reported that their menopause symptoms interfered with their lives; 42 percent of these women admitted they've never discussed menopause with their health care provider.[50] She-Who-Shall-Not-Be-Named, You Know Who, the Big "M" . . . let's stop treating menopause like Lord Voldemort and start talking about what comes after the reproductive years!

During the menopause transition, progesterone levels have already drastically dropped, and now estrogen levels begin to fluctuate. While progesterone tends to vanish like a flame in the wind, estrogen is a bit more stubborn, like the prank birthday candles that continue to relight after each attempt to blow them out. Much like a roller coaster, there are extreme highs and extreme lows, and levels can suddenly and unexpectedly change. It rages, it falls, it surges, then further skyrockets, plummets again, and what comes next is never quite certain. Progesterone supplementation may be helpful during the transition to menopause to balance the dramatic ups and downs of estrogen that occur.

After menopause, the ovaries retire from the hormone-making business and the adrenal glands take over. As a result, the menstrual cycle no longer occurs: no FSH/LH production, no preparing for pregnancy, no monthly bleed. Estrogen levels decline for good, finally tapering off to a lower but more steady level. Concerns over high levels of estrogen may now be a far distant memory. The hormonal imbalance associated with menopause is inadequate estrogen levels.

Lean body mass also declines with age, and, as energy expenditure decreases, weight gain is common. Paired with low estrogen levels, postmenopausal women begin to see more male-like fat patterning with adipose tissue increasing in the abdominal area instead of the hips and thighs. As discussed in chapter 4, it's now more critical than ever to eat adequate protein and incorporate some resistance training.

Now what to do about your hormone levels? Let them settle at their new, lower range without intervening. After all, this is a normal part of the aging process. But if you have negative symptoms, you may want to take action. There are two options to increase your estrogen levels, and the choice is yours to make. The first option is hormone replacement therapy. You'll need to work with your health care practitioner to dial in the appropriate plan if you choose this route. Hormone replacement therapy will effectively shut down the adrenal glands from making the sex hormones and provide a bioidentical supply, but, like most medications, this method is not without risks.

The other route is supplementing estrogens in your diet with phytoestrogens for a more natural approach to hormone balance. Phytoestrogens, such as soy, can provide relief for many negative symptoms of menopause and offer health benefits, including lowered risk of osteoporosis, heart disease, and breast cancer.[51] Phytoestrogens are plant compounds with estrogen-like properties; they can behave as estrogen in the body when naturally circulating levels of estrogen are low.[52] The problem with relying entirely on phytoestrogens for estrogen support on a standard

Keto-Friendly Phytoestrogens
- Low-carb soy products—tofu, soy sauce
- Sesame seeds
- Alfalfa sprouts
- Coffee
- Mint
- Lupin
- Flaxseed
- Almonds
- Sunflower seeds
- Olive oil

ketogenic diet is that many phytoestrogen sources are high in carbohydrates. There are low-carb phytoestrogens, but if you are seeking a wider variety of these plant-based estrogens in your diet, explore one of the alternative dieting strategies discussed in chapter 8.

Ketogenic diets can be an effective approach to dieting for postmenopausal women struggling with weight gain, but the diet can also provide neuroprotective benefits. Age and declining sex hormones after menopause are risk factors for Alzheimer's disease.[53] With epidemiological studies revealing two-thirds of Alzheimer's patients are female, it appears women are at higher risk for Alzheimer's disease than men.[54] Although Alzheimer's treatment is most certainly outside the scope of this book, it's worth a mention for those who may be affected by the disease. For more information about the therapeutic use of ketogenic diets for Alzheimer's disease, I highly recommend *The Alzheimer's Antidote* by Amy Berger.

Wonky Periods After Keto

If you start keto and *then* your periods go wild, what now? Relax! If you are using a ketogenic diet for weight loss, there are a couple things happening concurrently. One, your calories have been reduced, which can trigger a stress response in your body. Be honest: Are you cutting your calories too low? Are you really eating as much as you think you are? Ketogenic diets are appetite suppressing, which can be useful when trying to reduce calorie intake but can backfire if you aren't actually eating enough. Remember: The body sees undereating as a stressor; elevated cortisol will throttle your progesterone levels, and a missed period is a red flag to evaluate and adjust your calorie intake.

Another reason you could be experiencing erratic periods has to do with fat loss and the release of stored hormones and toxins. Adipose tissue is not just a storage space for fat—all kinds of things are stored here! They include fat-soluble vitamins, hormones, pollutants, toxins, and a variety of other substances that are foreign to the body.[55] While stored, they are slowly released into the bloodstream, but they are rapidly freed during weight loss as the fat deposits are burned for energy.[56] As these extra components enter the blood, your hormones and menstrual cycle may be affected. As we know, hormone balance is a delicate process, and even slight increases can trigger deviations in the system. Your body will either metabolize and excrete the excess that's been released or reabsorb it, so any imbalance this causes is only temporary. Ultimately you will be better off, as the pollutants in your body tend to decrease by about 15 percent after weight loss.[57] This also supports the argument for a slow and steady approach to fat loss, as you don't want to load your liver with an overabundance of toxins to metabolize all at once.[58]

Finally, a drop in carbohydrates has the potential to affect thyroid hormone production. For those susceptible to impaired thyroid function, this could also affect your menstrual cycle. We'll discuss thyroid hormones further in the next chapter, but I want to address it here for those with known thyroid issues. A dramatic drop in carbohydrates can undoubtedly affect your menstrual cycle, specifically if you are at risk of or have a thyroid-related disease. Beginning a keto diet doesn't have to be all or nothing; you don't have to go from high carb to no carb in the blink of an eye. Gradually ease into carbohydrate restriction if cutting carbohydrates quickly is problematic. You can also eat carbs strategically to counterbalance this effect, which will be discussed further in chapter 8. Listen to the clues your body gives you and adjust your approach accordingly.

Fertile Myrtle: Balanced Hormones and Keto Babies

If balanced hormones are indicative that our health is in good shape and our menstrual cycle is running like a well-oiled machine, then guess what? Your body is set up for reproductive success! If you want to get pregnant, this is undoubtedly the ideal state to be in. But if not, take precautions, such as the nonhormonal birth control methods mentioned previously (see page 75). Women with a history of menstrual dysfunction, absent or irregular periods, who start ovulating like clockwork can find themselves in for a big surprise!

There is plenty of anecdotal evidence for ketogenic diets increasing fertility levels—just do a quick Google search for "keto babies" or "keto got me pregnant" to find endless forums of women sharing their experience. But there's also solid research that shows that ketogenic diets can improve fertility in women by improving menstrual cyclicity, ovulation rates, and frequency of menses.[59] Weight loss in and of itself enhances fertility levels, but the additional benefits associated with ketogenic diets—reduced inflammation, improved mitochondrial function, and insulin sensitivity—may offer further fertility-enhancing benefits.[60] For women struggling with infertility, restoring your hormonal balance can also restore a bit of hope.

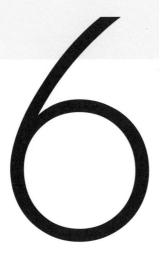

Oh, You Thought We Were Done with Hormones?

We've spent a great deal of time discussing the cyclical female hormones and the impact of hormonal imbalance. Now, let's dive into some of the other significant hormones that can affect your ability to lose body fat. That's right: Hormones can affect your body composition! Some of you may be thinking, "Wait, I thought you said calories were the most important thing when it comes to weight loss!" Guilty as charged, but hormones influence the energy balance in many ways; the two are intertwined in a sort of chicken-and-egg dilemma.

Hormones influence all systems in the body, affecting how much food you eat (calories in) and how much energy you burn (calories out). The macronutrient composition of the foods we eat (calories in) affects our hormones, which, in turn, drive our food intake (calories in) and energy expenditure (calories out). It's a big interconnected cycle, with energy balance (calories) and hormones closely linked in the system.

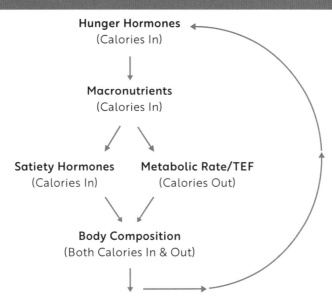

The relationship between hormones and energy balance is complex, but this flowchart provides a simplified visual of the most basic interactions.

We've already seen examples of this in the previous chapter, which explained how metabolic rate and energy intake are affected simply by hormonal changes of the menstrual cycle. Hormones have a significant impact on the good ol' "calories in, calories out" equation. But does that mean hormones are more important than calories when it comes to weight loss? No. Even with perfectly balanced hormones, if we eat at or above our energy needs, we will not lose weight. Hormones do not negate calorie balance, surplus, or deficit, but they do help regulate them. The take-home message is that when it comes to losing body fat, it's not exclusively calories or hormones—it's both.

Switching from sugar-burner to fat-burner gives us access to alternative metabolic pathways, and with this shift comes a fundamental change in our hormones. By manipulating "calories in" with a ketogenic diet, we can transform our hormonal state from one that hoards fat to one that readily burns it. We can now begin to explore how different hormones influence our metabolism and food intake and how keto can effectively shift the systems to work in our favor.

Nutritional ketosis brings on many hormonal changes that can positively affect our ability to lose body fat. The keto diet can be a useful tool for weight loss, as the hormonal changes brought on by carbohydrate restriction affect our hunger levels, ability to store body fat, and even metabolic rate. Instead of blaming our hormones for causing us to overeat (calories in) or for our sluggish metabolisms (calories out), we can change how we fuel the body with a keto diet (calories in), which will trigger a domino effect of positive hormonal responses that can be used to benefit our body composition. It's not all sunshine and roses, though; as we'll see, there are certain situations in which the hormonal shift may bring about undesirable or less than ideal effects, which can be addressed with minor adjustments and dieting strategies that fall outside the realm of a standard ketogenic diet.

The Hormone Factory: Endocrine System and Adipose Tissue

Hormone production is handled by the endocrine system, a collection of endocrine glands. Often called the "master gland," the pituitary gland serves as the control center for all the other endocrine glands. These glands manufacture hormones with specific functions, such as energy metabolism or reproduction. They include the pituitary, pineal, thyroid, thymus, adrenals, pancreas, and ovaries in women. The hypothalamus and pituitary run the show, gauging hormonal levels and sending out signals to the endocrine glands throughout the body. The endocrine glands respond to the commands, either ramping up production of a hormone or turning it off.

Think of the interaction between the hypothalamus, pituitary, and endocrine glands like the NASA Mission Control Center giving directions to astronauts in their spacecraft, who then give feedback to Earth.

One thing you might not expect is that the hypothalamus also interacts with body fat. For a long time, many scientists believed that adipose tissue was simply storage space, but we now know adipose tissue is a tremendous player in our endocrine system.[1] In addition to providing a reservoir for body fat, vitamins, xenobiotics, and toxins, adipose tissue is also its own little hormone factory, actively manufacturing and secreting a variety of bioactive molecules. Much like the endocrine glands, adipose tissue produces chemical messengers—estrogen, leptin, resistin, cytokines—that participate in the regulation of sugar and fat metabolism, energy balance, feeding behavior, insulin sensitivity, inflammation, and creation of new fat cells.[2] Unlike the endocrine glands, adipose tissue continues to grow, and the cells keep multiplying, skewing the hormonal contribution of the tissue and dramatically affecting the rest of the body. The quantity of adipose tissue affects the production of these hormones and chemical messengers to the point that obesity is synonymous with hormonal imbalance and inflammation.

By lowering our body fat levels, we are promoting healthy hormonal balance and reducing inflammatory factors. Obesity is a clear sign that body systems are off-kilter; the longer we carry the extra weight, and the higher our body fat levels climb, the more out of whack things end up leading to insulin resistance, type 2 diabetes, cardiovascular disease, and more. Losing body fat can help restore balance.

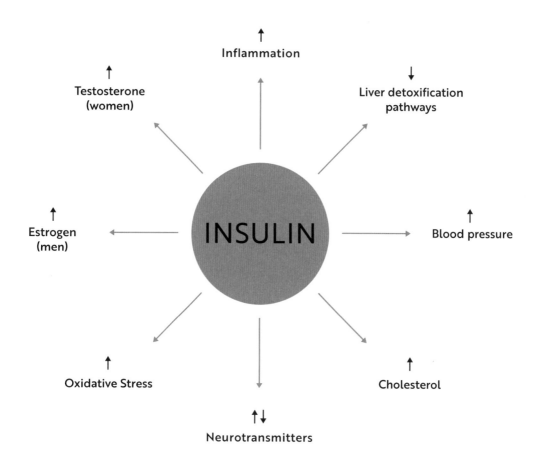

Insulin: The Storage Hormone

Insulin, as we've discussed, is a storage hormone; when blood sugar becomes high, insulin is secreted by the pancreas to help stabilize glucose levels in the bloodstream. After a meal, blood glucose rises and insulin levels follow, which signals cells to sweep in nutrients. Excess glucose is cleared from the blood and fatty acids are taken in by adipose tissue for storage until needed for fuel. In the fed state, when insulin levels are highest, the body is in storage mode; not all nutrients brought in with a meal will be used immediately, so the body wants to hang on to them for when energy is needed later. Glucose is converted into its stored form, glycogen, and fatty acids are stored as triacylglycerols in adipose tissue.

This is one reason that quickly digested foods, such as sugar and other refined carbohydrates, are best avoided when trying to avoid excess storage. Rather than a slow and steady supply of nutrients that gradually raise blood sugar and insulin, which provides prolonged support of energy needs, the body is presented with a rapid influx of energy that can either be burned right away or stored for later use. These quick bursts of fuel exceed the body's demands in most scenarios, and the surplus of energy heads off to storage. Higher glycemic index (GI) foods tend to rapidly digest and absorb, providing a sharp increase in blood glucose and insulin levels; lower GI foods have slower digestion periods, effecting a more gradual rise in glucose and insulin.[3]

Immediately following a meal, when insulin levels are at their height, the breakdown of stored fat for energy is inhibited. Why would the body need to break down stored energy when there are plenty of nutrients readily flowing through the bloodstream? It's not until insulin levels fall between meals that stored glycogen or triacylglycerols are burned for energy, as nutrients in the blood become scarce.

Insulin for Strength Training

Of course, insulin isn't all doom and gloom. Insulin also promotes preservation of muscle tissue by preventing muscle from being degraded.[4] If you are actively trying to build muscle, then insulin's actions can certainly work in your favor. This is one of the downfalls of a ketogenic diet, in that insulin is conducive to muscle growth and recovery.[5] If you are interested in bodybuilding or strength training, you will often hear that low-carb diets are a poor pairing. Rest assured, there are ways of working around this, as we'll discuss in chapter 8. For those looking to increase lean body mass while eating a ketogenic diet, strategically spiking insulin levels around workouts can help counter this potential disadvantage.

We can keep insulin levels lower by reducing the incoming quick-digesting carbohydrates and limiting our food intake while being mindful of energy balance. When we maintain chronically high insulin levels, our body doesn't get a break from storage mode; body fat isn't burned for energy while we're shoveling more and more fatty acids into storage. This is the scenario we create when overeating, which can quickly lead to weight gain. This is also the road to insulin resistance (see page 39).

Ketogenic diets are famous for reducing insulin levels. Through carbohydrate restriction, we can stop stoking the blood-sugar fire that drives those levels up. The drop in insulin levels allows access to fat stores for energy burn, helps alleviate insulin resistance, and gives an overtaxed pancreas a much-needed break. For those looking to achieve fat loss, this is ideal.

Ways to Improve Insulin Resistance

- Limit carbohydrate intake or eat high-fiber, low-glycemic carbs
- Eat anti-inflammatory foods
- Decrease body fat
- Exercise!

The insulin hormone often gets a bad rap. Just ask type 1 diabetics whether insulin is all bad; unable to produce adequate levels of insulin, they rely on insulin therapy to manage their condition. Insulin is important, but too much or too little can have a negative effect. It's all about balance.

When the balance has been thrown off, it is more often an issue of too much insulin, or *hyperinsulinemia*. This condition is accompanied by insulin resistance, or impaired sensitivity to the insulin hormone, which one-third of the adult population in the United States suffers from.[6] Many factors contribute to insulin resistance, including obesity and inflammation, which go hand in hand with imbalanced hormones. Even menstruation can affect our sensitivity to insulin, as we tend to be more sensitive to insulin in the first phase of the cycle and lose this sensitivity as insulin resistance rears its ugly head during the later luteal phase.

How can we lessen insulin resistance? Removing or decreasing incoming factors that contribute to desensitization of insulin is a good place to start. A ketogenic diet is certainly one way to do this, but if you are easing into carbohydrate restriction, focus on removing quickly digested simple sugars and refined carbs from your diet. Inflammation is also a major contributing factor to insulin resistance; while reducing body fat will certainly reduce inflammation, focusing on eating anti-inflammatory foods and reducing inflammatory foods can boost insulin sensitivity. Last, but certainly not least, incorporating exercise into your lifestyle can greatly lessen insulin sensitivity. Both anaerobic and aerobic exercise have been found to lessen insulin sensitivity significantly.

A calorie-conscious ketogenic diet can be used as a tool to attack insulin resistance from several angles: promotion of low insulin, reduced body fat, and anti-inflammatory effects. Pair that with your favorite choice of physical activity and kiss insulin resistance goodbye!

Hungry, Hungry Hormones: Appetite and Feeding Behavior

Between meals, when your stomach is empty, it creates the hormone ghrelin. Ghrelin is one of the only hormones known to stimulate the appetite—it sends messages to the hypothalamus to start shoveling food into your mouth.

Once you eat, ghrelin levels fall. However, not all macronutrients are created equal when it comes to decreasing those levels. Highly refined carbohydrates, such as high-fructose corn syrup, can impair ghrelin's response.[7] Protein, however, can reduce ghrelin levels, which is one reason why it is the most satiating macronutrient.[8] Another way to ensure ghrelin levels drop? Eating a keto diet, of course! Ketogenic diets have a ghrelin-suppressing effect, which explains their hunger-curbing benefits.[9]

Ghrelin levels usually increase with weight loss. As you lose body fat, your body tries to fight back and ramps up production of ghrelin. As a result, you become hungrier and hungrier. It's an uphill battle to maintain weight loss—how can you keep your new, lower energy balance if you are fighting against your body's demands to eat, eat, eat?!

Fortunately, ketogenic diets outshine traditional calorie restriction when it comes to managing hunger. Studies have shown that ghrelin levels do not increase during weight loss while in ketosis.[10] Instead, nutritional ketosis inhibits the ghrelin hormone. You can use a ketogenic diet to weaken the grip that ghrelin has on your appetite and hunger. This can allow you to make serious progress and retain it. Many people (myself included) will tell you that the best diet is the one that you stick to; in my experience, the lack of voracious hunger helps.

Decreased hunger is hands down one of the reasons keto diets can be so useful for people looking to lose weight and keep it off. In fact, many studies have attributed weight loss on a ketogenic diet with a spontaneous reduction in calorie intake.[11] Without instruction to restrict or count calories, overweight and obese individuals naturally cut back on their incoming energy while in nutritional ketosis. A calorie deficit doesn't come from the practice of tracking or counting calories; it's a result of eating less. Ketogenic diets are a great way to encourage your body to take in less energy voluntarily—fantastic for the women who thrive with intuitive eating or have no interest in tallying food-related numbers.

Why Do You Stop Eating?

As food travels through your digestive tract, hormones are released to help regulate your appetite. When nutrients reach their landmarks along the way, appetite-suppressing hormones are unleashed. For example, when food leaves the stomach to enter the small intestine, the amino acids, partially digested proteins, and fats trigger the release of cholecystokinin (CCK), a hormone that suppresses the appetite. Glucagon-like peptide (GLP-1) and peptide YY (PYY) are also released as nutrients travel the length of the intestine. These two hormones slow the rate of food leaving the stomach and pump the brakes on intestinal motility, factors that reduce the speed digested food travels through the gut and contribute to satiety.

All this has quite a lot to do with gastric emptying rates—how quickly food leaves your stomach. Food's macronutrient composition also plays a huge role in this process. As a general rule, the faster the stomach is emptied, the fewer appetite-suppressing hormones are released. And remember, an empty stomach produces ghrelin. Gastric emptying rates also affect the glucose-insulin response previously mentioned in this chapter. Quickly digested food, such as simple sugars and other refined carbohydrates, rapidly exit the stomach and are then absorbed via the small intestine. In addition to spiking blood sugar and insulin, the rushed rate at which this occurs leads to less exposure to the nutrients in the gut that prompt the release of PYY, GLP-1, and CCK.

Speaking of CCK, proteins and fats are primarily responsible for triggering the release of this hormone, not carbohydrates—yet another reason these macronutrients tend to be more sating. Slowly digested food, such as protein, fats, and fiber, drag down gastric emptying rates. This creates a slow and steady drip of nutrients exiting the stomach into the small intestine. In turn, if the amount of time CCK, GLP-1, and PYY are secreted is maximized, their levels are increased, and their impact is prolonged. Lower glycemic index foods also promote satiety by way of a slower rate of gastric emptying and extended CCK production.[12] This is why something purely sugary, such as a huge soda or a bag of hard candy, won't fill you up and satisfy your hunger, while a relatively small amount of steak or chicken breast will usually do the trick.

The Role of Sex Hormones in Hunger and Appetite

Recall from the last chapter: At the end of each monthly cycle, women can experience increased appetite and ravenous cravings that cause them to eat hundreds of extra calories during the luteal phase. Those of us interested in losing weight probably want to know why the heck that happens and how to prevent it.

There are significant variations in appetite and energy intake during the menstrual cycle, which can, in part, be explained by the influence of estrogen and progesterone on the digestive process and hormones. As estrogen and progesterone levels rise and fall on a cyclical basis, so do the gastric emptying rates.

During the estrogen-dominant follicular phase—the first part of the cycle, when insulin sensitivity is high and energy intake tends to be balanced—food leaves the stomach at a slower rate.[13] You feel satisfied after eating, you stay full for longer periods between meals, and as a result, you don't overeat.

During the progesterone-driven luteal phase—the later part of the cycle synonymous with desensitized insulin response, wild food cravings, and increased calorie intake—gastric emptying rates speed up.[14] Stomachs that are quickly emptied are stomachs that will soon be growling with hunger. During this period, you are left feeling hungry between meals and tend to overeat. We also know that cravings kick in during this time.[15] Indulging these cravings with sugary, high-carb sweets further drives quick transit through the stomach and prevents the appetite-suppressing hormones from doing their job.

Knowing we can alter the digestive process of gastric emptying with simple tweaks to the macronutrient composition of our foods, we can conclude a ketogenic approach would diminish the tendency to overeat during the luteal phase of the menstrual cycle.

Obesity and Hunger Hormones

In women who are obese, hunger and appetite-regulating hormones don't typically behave as expected. Rather than dramatically falling after a meal, ghrelin levels only slightly decrease after eating in these individuals.[16] With uninterrupted high levels of ghrelin, overeating continues to be problematic. Pair this with increasing ghrelin levels that accompany traditional weight loss efforts, and it is no wonder obesity is so difficult to overcome. Using ketogenic diets to reach a healthy weight can help restore standard ghrelin response without the added obstacle of fighting the counterproductive increased ghrelin levels associated with weight loss. Obese individuals also have lower levels of circulating appetite-suppressing GLP-1 and PYY hormones, but weight loss can restore healthy levels.[17]

What if your stomach doesn't empty its contents into the small intestine? What if rather than a rapid exit or slow drip there is a total delay? When this happens, the hormones that trigger you to stop eating aren't released on time, and you continue to eat well beyond your energy needs.[18] In women with delayed gastric emptying, it takes longer for the stomach to start releasing the nutrients and, in turn, longer for the cues to stop eating to take effect. This is seen in women with a history of obesity, binge eating, and bulimia.[19]

With repeated binges, stomach capacity can increase in size, taking longer to fill and, consequently, delaying the release of nutrients and postponing the release of appetite-suppressing hormones such as CCK.[20] Scientists J. D. Latner and G. T. Wilson[21] explored the effects of macronutrient intake on satiety in bulimia nervosa and found that increased protein intake decreased binge-eating episodes and was accompanied by a higher release of the CCK hormone and improved satiety signals. Their findings suggest that modifying the

Indulging these cravings with sugary, high-carb sweets further drives quick transit through the stomach and prevents the appetite-suppressing hormones from doing their job.

Leptin Resistance and Weight Gain: A Vicious Cycle

Gain Weight
Leptin levels and number of fat cells increase as fat is gained.

Increased Calorie Intake
Hunger persists despite increased calorie intake, leading to weight gain.

Leptin Resistance
Resistance to leptin develops as fat stores and inflammation increase.

Overeating
Food cravings and overeating are triggered by low leptin levels.

Disrupted Signal
Although there are abundant levels of stored fat and leptin, leptin's signal to the brain is disrupted and not received.

Leaky Gut Syndrome

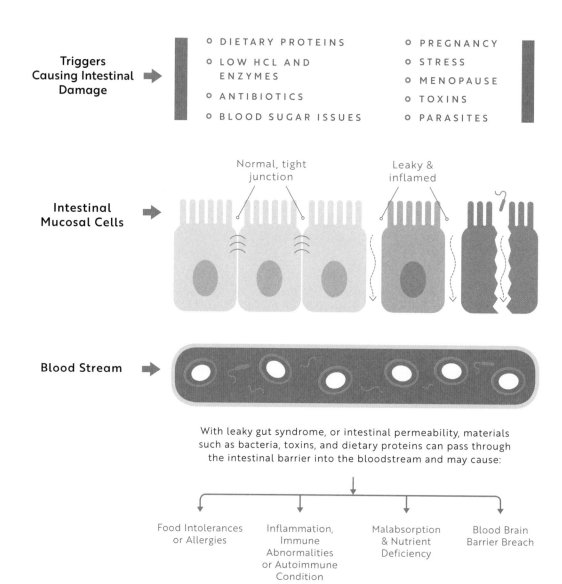

Triggers Causing Intestinal Damage

- DIETARY PROTEINS
- LOW HCL AND ENZYMES
- ANTIBIOTICS
- BLOOD SUGAR ISSUES

- PREGNANCY
- STRESS
- MENOPAUSE
- TOXINS
- PARASITES

Intestinal Mucosal Cells

Normal, tight junction

Leaky & inflamed

Blood Stream

With leaky gut syndrome, or intestinal permeability, materials such as bacteria, toxins, and dietary proteins can pass through the intestinal barrier into the bloodstream and may cause:

Food Intolerances or Allergies

Inflammation, Immune Abnormalities or Autoimmune Condition

Malabsorption & Nutrient Deficiency

Blood Brain Barrier Breach

macronutrient composition of meals may serve as an effective strategy for binge-eating behaviors.[22] By focusing on eating food with highly satiating macronutrients—protein, fat, and fiber—we can help counter the effects of delayed gastric emptying.

One crucial hormone I've yet to discuss is leptin, which is produced by fat cells. Leptin is a satiety hormone that helps regulate energy balance. As adipose tissue expands, increasing numbers of fat cells are available to create the leptin hormone; leptin sends off signals that energy stores are plentiful and large amounts of food intake are not needed. When functional, this communication mechanism between leptin and the hypothalamus serves to match food intake with energy needs.

As you would expect, higher levels of body fat are associated with higher levels of leptin. In theory, increased leptin levels should lead to decreased eating. And with regard to obesity, this overabundance of leptin should trigger a screaming alarm to your body to stop taking in more fuel. But when it comes to obesity, the leptin mechanism is broken. Much like we see with insulin resistance, the body's response to leptin is impaired. Rather than receiving signals that we have a copious bounty of energy stored in adipose tissue, the body reacts as though there is none. This is known as leptin resistance.[23] United with decreased levels of appetite-suppressing hormones and faulty postmeal ghrelin response, leptin resistance drives obese individuals to eat in excess even though their bodies don't need the energy.

Leptin resistance is linked to chronically high levels of insulin and inflammation.[24] The same steps to improve insulin resistance, lower insulin levels, and relieve inflammation can be used to repair the broken leptin mechanism. As we've learned, ketogenic diets can be a very effective way to achieve this. A calorie-restricted ketogenic diet can be used to lose excess body fat, which will also improve how the body responds to leptin.

Hormonal Balance Takes Guts: Microbiota and Intestinal Health

There are many cases in nature in which two species team up to help each other out: bees and flowers, clownfish and sea anemones, crocodiles and plover birds. Humans and bacteria are such a pair—and an often-overlooked piece of our hormonal balance puzzle. Inside our intestinal tract is a community of bacteria hanging out, living in harmony with our body. These colonies help us digest food, protect us from pathogens, and produce vitamins—they even help us metabolize hormones.

Find Out More on Binge Eating

While hormones can certainly contribute to binge eating, the behavior has a colossal psychological component to it that's outside the scope of this book or ketogenic diets. For strategies to help overcome binge eating, I highly recommend the books *Brain over Binge* by Kathryn Hansen and *The Little Book of Big Change* by Amy Johnson.

When we eat poor diets, our friendly bacteria become compromised and harmful bacteria can better compete for the territory. As a result, we can end up with pathogenic bacteria or an overgrowth of an individual species. Lacking the full range of diversity required for healthy, flourishing bacterial colonies, we lose some of the critical functionality our microbial friends provide.

Rather than bacterial colonies that benefit our bodies, we become hosts to microorganisms that hog our resources, impede our ability to absorb vitamins and nutrients properly, weaken our immune systems, and contribute to an inflammatory environment. A shift from good to bad bacteria, or an overgrowth of any particular species, can also affect our bodies' ability to metabolize hormones such as estrogens, testosterone, and cortisol.[25]

When the bacteria in our guts become unbalanced—this is known as dysbiosis—our hormones follow suit. Each individual strain of bacteria has its own role in the system; if one species runs rampant or is completely wiped out, the functional impact the organism has on hormones can either be amplified or silenced. Gut dysbiosis will contribute to hormonal imbalance.

Gut dysbiosis can also lead to inflammation and increased intestinal permeability.[27] Think of the intestine as a long tube lined with tightly packed cells that act as gatekeepers to the bloodstream and the rest of the body. These cells facilitate what comes into the body during the absorptive process of digestion, but they also act as barriers to prevent unwanted pathogens, debris, and partially digested molecules from entering. When these tight junctions between the intestinal cells become loose, intestinal permeability increases, and some things that aren't supposed to be taken in by the body leak into the bloodstream. This triggers an immune response, and the body goes to work attacking these foreign invaders; that's great if these are genuinely harmful things leaking in, but it can be a problem when the body starts attacking partially digested nutrients from a recently eaten meal. This phenomenon is known as leaky gut syndrome and is thought to be the cause of inflammation and many autoimmune diseases.

The loose junctions of the intestinal wall represent damage to the structural integrity of the intestine and can be caused by more than imbalanced microbial gut flora. Food allergens are a well-known contributor to increased intestinal permeability. One of the most widely known examples is gluten, with the protein causing structural damage to the intestine in those who are allergic or sensitive, triggering a subsequent inflammatory response as the protein enters the bloodstream.[28]

Other contributing factors can cause intestinal damage that leads to loose junctions between intestinal cells: antibiotics, high sugar intake, hormonal birth control, stress, insulin resistance, parasites, toxins, menopause, pregnancy, and the list goes on and on. The point is that our guts are extremely sensitive to what we put into our bodies. The best thing we can

How chronic stress can make you fat

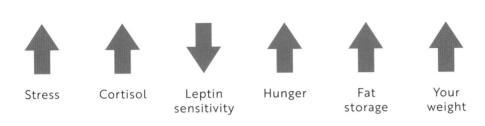

| Stress | Cortisol | Leptin sensitivity | Hunger | Fat storage | Your weight |

*Adapted from: Hyman, M. 2006. *Ultrametabolism*, 115. New Your, NY: Scribner.

do to prevent damage and begin healing the gut is to eliminate foods that are inflammatory to us and restore balance to our microbial friends.

To fix our guts, first, we need to fix our diets. Avoiding highly refined carbohydrates and sugar, eliminating potential allergens, and eating nutrient-dense foods are excellent ways to start. Probiotics, prebiotics, and fermented foods with live cultures are a great way to reintroduce healthy, diverse microbial populations back into your system.[29]

Let's Talk about Stress, Baby

Stress can affect your hormonal health and metabolism. Cortisol is a hormone produced by your adrenal glands and released in response to stress. As part of the fight-or-flight response, cortisol's job is to act against insulin and keep glucose in the bloodstream for quick energy. To ensure high levels of blood sugar are available for fast fuel, cortisol impairs glucose uptake into cells while stimulating gluconeogenesis in the liver.[30] In an emergency, like a bear chasing you, a quick burst of cortisol and instant access to energy could give you the fuel to get out of immediate danger! Once the threat passes, your hormones go back to normal.

So what's the problem? In our modern society, the stressors come from all angles. We aren't usually chased by animals, but the agonizing commute to work, the endless deadlines, the toxic relationships, the bills, and [insert your biggest stressor here] all contribute to increased cortisol levels. Our bodies are left to produce cortisol nonstop. Chronic stress and elevated cortisol levels go hand in hand.

As a result, your hormone balance can be thrown entirely out of whack. High cortisol can lead to low progesterone and interrupt the menstrual cycle, which we briefly touched on in the previous chapter. Without progesterone to balance the estrogens, we have yet another example of how estrogens can quickly dominate a hormonal imbalance.

Chronically high cortisol levels can also contribute to insulin resistance and the development of type 2 diabetes.[31] With cortisol continuously working against insulin's actions, the body is left with high blood glucose levels and increased insulin production. The cycle continues until it can't any longer. High insulin levels contribute to increased fat storage, weight gain, and decreased sensitivity to the effects of insulin.

Elevated cortisol can also cause dramatic amounts of water retention.[32] Although a natural fluctuation of water weight is normal, severe water retention can lead to dangerously high blood pressure and abdominal obesity.[33]

As you can see, your emotional and physical well-being affect your hormone balance. In addition to emotional stress, your body interprets many things as stressors—injury, illness, lack of sleep, trauma. Many factors can contribute to the incoming stress load, including our diets.

When it comes to our diet, a severe drop in carb and calorie intake can also trigger a stress response. Scientist Mohorko and his colleagues[34] investigated the hormonal response of obese women losing weight on a twelve-week calorie-restricted ketogenic diet. Despite improvements in nearly all hormonal parameters, weight loss, improved cognitive function, and physical performance, the women experienced increased cortisol levels for the duration of the study.[35] The take-home: Restricting carbohydrates and calories can be interpreted as stress by the body.

Does that mean you shouldn't try the keto diet? Nope. *Any* diet will have a similar effect. Calorie restriction, regardless of how it's achieved, will lead to elevated cortisol. We know if you want to lose weight, a calorie deficit is necessary. So, what should we do? First, we can embrace the idea of a moderate calorie deficit and resist the urge to drop our intake dramatically. The next step is doing your best to eliminate the other stressors in your life or finding a way to process them. Don't underestimate the power of mental health and self-care! Get a good night's sleep, meditate, do yoga, take a walk, head to the gym, start a journal, blast your music, dance, paint a picture, call a close friend, spend time in the garden, take a nice bath, scream into a pillow . . . just chill! Whatever healthy form of stress relief you find works for you, keep it up. It will pay off in dividends.

> "In a world of stressful lack of control, an amazing source of control we all have is the ability to make the world a better place, one act at a time."
>
> —Robert M. Sapolsky, *Why Zebras Don't Get Ulcers: The Acclaimed Guide to Stress, Stress-Related Diseases, and Coping*

Thyroid: Can You Even Do Keto?

Did you know that the butterfly-shaped thyroid gland in your neck is responsible for regulating the metabolism of the millions of cells throughout your body? The rate at which each cell burns fuel is largely influenced by the thyroid hormones, another set of chemical messengers. The two primary hormones produced and secreted by the thyroid gland are T3 (triiodothyronine) and T4 (thyroxine). T3 is the more biologically active form of the hormone, though T4 can be converted to T3 as needed.

Thyroid status correlates with body weight and energy expenditure—increased levels are associated with a sped-up metabolism via increased caloric burn and weight loss; decreased levels are associated with a slowed metabolic rate, reduced energy expenditure, and weight gain.[36] Fluctuation in the thyroid hormones can cause either an increase or decrease in metabolic rate, which can affect your ability to lose weight. Imagine fueling up your vehicle and pressing down on the gas to move forward, but, even when you floor it, your car slowly inches down the street instead of zooming off toward the horizon. This is what it is like to have low thyroid levels, an inefficient engine to burn your full tank of gas.

The paradox we so often see when dieting is active thyroid levels drop. During periods when we're restricting calorie intake, our body wants to slow down how much energy it burns and hold on to what it has. It's another adaptive trait to keep us alive and thriving during times when food is scarce, but a potentially annoying mechanism when you are trying to lose weight. Our active thyroid levels drop as a result of the lower calorie intake, and our metabolic rate adapts. Once we increase our food intake, our thyroid levels bounce back.

For a woman with a normal functioning thyroid, this tends to be more annoying than problematic. But the truth of the matter is many women have underlying thyroid issues, most commonly an underactive thyroid, or hypothyroidism.[37] Even before beginning a diet, their metabolic rates aren't running at optimal speed, and, as a result, their bodies don't burn as many calories.

There are a variety of reasons for this, some of which are genetic,[38] but often they are hormonal. Excess estrogen can decrease free levels of T4 and T3 while simultaneously suppressing the conversion of T4 to the active T3.[39] In this case, what appears to be thyroid dysfunction is actually a hormone imbalance. We know when it comes to hormonal imbalance, high levels of estrogens tend to be the most prevalent disruptor.[40] The common imbalance in women is becoming clearer: high estrogens, low thyroid, trouble managing weight. Correcting the hormonal balance at the estrogen level has the potential to improve thyroid function.

Knowing a drop in calories also causes active thyroid levels to drop, many women with underactive thyroid or low thyroid hormone levels are advised not to cut calories. There is also some evidence that carbohydrate restriction reduces the active form T3 as well.[41] Because of this, the use of low-carb diets for women with existing thyroid issues is controversial,

The Experts Weigh In

Ketogenic diets can be quite a polarizing topic when it comes to thyroid health; there are experts on both sides of the argument. Just like any good controversy, there are those who vehemently oppose and those who rally to support. The truth is, it's difficult to know without more evidence-based research; studies involving ketogenic diets and impaired thyroid are still largely uncharted territory.

Among experts who support the use of ketogenic diets for women with thyroid issues is doctor and researcher Stephen Phinney, MD, PhD. Phinney[42] has proposed that the body becomes more sensitive to thyroid hormones after following a ketogenic diet, similar to the increased insulin sensitivity observed.[43] As a result, the drop in thyroid hormone levels may actually be negligent as our body becomes more responsive to the lower circulating levels. The shift in thyroid levels during carbohydrate restriction could represent a "new normal" when the body is operating within the physiological conditions of nutritional ketosis.

Dr. Cate Shanahan also supports the use of low-carb diets in this context but advises dieters to ease gradually into carbohydrate restriction.[44] Shanahan suggests that a rapid decrease in carbohydrates may trigger a reflex in some women that interferes with the pathway of converting T4 to active T3. Women with thyroid concerns may be able to avoid the effects of lower active thyroid hormone by slowly transitioning into carbohydrate restriction instead of diving right in.

to say the least. Working with your health care practitioner to correct low thyroid levels *before* reducing calories or carbs would be the most ideal scenario for those concerned with hypothyroidism. Hormone replacement therapy may be necessary. Then you can work together to adjust treatment once you begin a diet—whether it is keto or something else is up to you and your doctor.

If thyroid health is a concern, but you have your heart set on trying the keto diet for its known benefits, consider the possibility of transitioning into a low-carb diet. Rather than dramatically cutting carbs in the beginning, ease into it. Start by lowering little by little each day and see how you feel. If you get to ketogenic levels and your body is screaming at you to quit (and your electrolytes are in check—more on this in chapter 12), then ease off. Listen to your body.

My second suggestion is to try alternating periods of extended calorie and carbohydrate restriction followed by planned carbohydrate refeeds and/or increased calorie intake. Taking planned breaks from calorie restriction to allow your thyroid hormone levels to rebound can be an effective way to signal to your body that you aren't actually in a famine. Periodically increasing your carbohydrate intake can also have positive effects on your hormones and metabolism. Cyclical ketogenic diets may very well have a place in your life!

Anecdotally, some women with impaired thyroid function choose to forgo carb refeeds and report no ill effect. Does that mean I recommend it? Not quite. It's up to you and your health care provider to determine what is appropriate in your situation. Most of the time, health complications such as this are not as simple as a quick macronutrient adjustment to set things on the right path. Based on the current literature, I suggest steering clear of dramatically reducing carbs right away and embracing the idea of cycling carbs once you become fat-adapted. Remember, there is nothing inherently wrong with carbohydrates. If you are unable to follow a standard ketogenic diet, there are other ways.

CH 7

Exercise and Athletic Training

One thing many women worry about when transitioning to a low-carb lifestyle is how it will affect their workouts. At rest, our brain is the primary energy hog, but when physical activity is increased, energy requirements for working muscles explode. Current sports dietary guidelines and traditional knowledge surrounding exercise support high carbohydrate intake—but can nutritional ketosis handle the job?

The quick answer: Yes. You absolutely can fuel your workouts sans carbs. However, there may be scenarios in which strategically using carbohydrates can complement your efforts. In this chapter, we'll gain a better understanding of the role of exercise in fat loss and explore the pros and cons of ketogenic diets for exercise and athletic training.

Exercise and Fat Loss

If you are using keto as a tool to burn body fat, I strongly recommend incorporating some form of physical activity into your routine. Here's why.

We burn calories during exercise. The first and, perhaps, most obvious reason to include exercise in your plan is that you burn more calories during physical activity as the body's energy demands increase. Even small amounts of physical activity can add up to substantial amounts over time. In the grand scheme of energy balance, being more active will work in your favor.

Exercise protects lean body mass. Staying physically active is imperative to the preservation of lean tissue throughout our lives. Loss of lean mass is a very real risk that commonly accompanies dieting and weight loss, but physical activity can help prevent this. Both endurance and strength training have been found to combat the loss of lean tissue that comes with aging in women.[1] Furthermore, resistance training can help efforts to increase or maintain lean body mass for women while simultaneously supporting fat loss efforts on ketogenic diets.[2] Remember, when losing weight, our focus is to reduce body fat, not muscle.

Exercise can increase BMR. Certain types of exercise even have the potential to boost your metabolism, independent of changes in body composition. In one recent study, researchers placed sedentary adult women on a novice resistance-training program for six weeks and, at the end of the study, observed significant improvements to their basal metabolic rates (BMR).[3] Think back to chapter 4: The BMR is the bare minimum amount of calories burned to keep your body functioning lying entirely still. Simply by participating in some form of resistance training, the number of calories your body burns will increase, even at rest, outside of calories burned during physical activity.

Exercise improves insulin sensitivity. While physical inactivity has been linked to insulin resistance, exercise has been proven to improve insulin sensitivity and glucose homeostasis dramatically.[4] The energy demands mediated through muscle contraction elicit a response to usher in glucose, independent of insulin's actions.[5] By simply moving more, we can improve the way our bodies respond to carbohydrates. We know that ketogenic diets also do a fantastic job addressing insulin resistance. The combination of keto and exercise can be an effective way to alleviate the insulin resistance that plagues a considerable portion of the population.

Physical activity relieves stress. It is well known that many people use exercise as an outlet for stress relief. For those who enjoy working out, a regular exercise routine can be a useful tool for coping with the stressors that crop up in our daily lives. Chronic stress can lead to an overproduction of the cortisol hormone and dysregulation of hormonal systems, as discussed in chapter 6. Physical activity has been proven to improve the brain-adrenal response and buffer the effects of stress.[6] This is good news for those of us with chronically high cortisol levels impeding hormonal balance and weight loss efforts.

Exercise improves anabolic hormones. As we age, our sex hormones take a dive, and, as a result, our lean body mass dwindles. Both endurance and resistance exercise elicit an acute hormonal response that benefits maintenance and improvements in lean body mass. Copeland et al.[7] found that physical activity increased the anabolic (muscle-building) hormone levels—estradiol, testosterone, growth hormone, DHEA—in women up to sixty-nine years old (the age of the oldest participant).[8] Exercise can be a fantastic way for women to maintain functional capacity and preserve lean body mass as we age. This will help us keep our metabolic rate up and battle the weight gain commonly experienced in menopausal and postmenopausal years.

Keto and Exercise: The One-Two Punch

Combining a ketogenic diet with exercise can give extra body fat the one-two punch while supercharging your quest for hormonal balance. Though exercise is not a mandatory element for fat loss, it can undoubtedly accelerate it.

Dr. Jeff Volek[9] led a study comparing the effects of resistance training on low-carb and low-fat diets on overweight individuals.[10] The resistancetraining groups performed three days a week and were evaluated against the nontraining groups. Not surprisingly, the group combining a keto diet with resistance training lost the most body fat among all the other training and diet groups:

- **Keto + Resistance Training:** 5.3 percent reduction in body fat
- **Low Fat + Resistance Training:** 3.5 percent reduction in body fat
- **Keto + No Exercise:** 3.4 percent reduction in body fat
- **Low Fat + No Exercise:** 2 percent reduction in body fat[11]

This study shows that in addition to preserving lean body mass, resistance training can drive fat loss and significantly improve results. Combining a keto diet with some form of resistance training is an ideal strategy for optimal fat loss.

Your diet alone will deliver the majority of the results, but adding exercise to the mix will help protect your muscles, accelerate your progress, and provide a healthy outlet for stress management. Aside from what we've discussed, the benefits of physical activity extend well beyond aesthetics and body composition. If you don't currently exercise, it is something to consider seriously.

Fuel Usage during Exercise

When carb intake is high, carbohydrates are the human body's preferred fuel source. As sugar pumps through your bloodstream, your body has instant access to energy. This energy is quickly depleted by the increased energy demands of exercise, and the body turns to its energy stores: glycogen and body fat.

The amount of energy stored in glycogen is much less than what is stored in our adipose tissue. While our fat storage is endless, glycogen storage is limited. In a carb-fueled individual,

Which Fuel Tank Would you Choose?

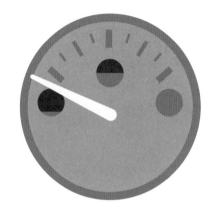

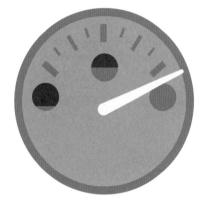

2,000Kcal

> 40,000Kcal

GLYCOGEN TANK

FAT TANK

Once your body becomes fully adapted to using fat as its preferred fuel, your brain and muscles no longer have to compete for suitable fuel.

this can be problematic during long periods of endurance exercise. As glycogen levels become depleted during a workout, the fuel source becomes low and requires replenishment in individuals who are not efficient at burning fat for fuel. This is known as "hitting the wall," when overwhelming fatigue and loss of energy sets in during endurance exercise.

If your body is used to fueling with carbohydrates and your glycogen tank runs low, your brain and actively working muscles end up competing for limited glucose produced from noncarbohydrate sources via gluconeogenesis instead.[12]

In the initial stages of carbohydrate restriction, there is often a period of reduced performance as the body adjusts to the ketogenic metabolic pathway.[13] The glycogen tank is running on empty right out of the gate, and while your body is always able to use fat for fuel, developing an efficient fat-burning metabolism takes several weeks of low-carb dieting. The time required to become fat-adapted tends to reflect a period of decreased athletic performance, so don't expect to set any personal records immediately after starting keto.

The good news is, impaired performance is only temporary. Once your body becomes fully adapted to using fat as its preferred fuel, your brain and muscles no longer have to compete for suitable fuel during prolonged bouts of exercise. Brain cells can meet energy demands with ketones while the muscles burn a mix of fatty acids and ketones—an adaptation that can effectively shield you from the effects of "hitting the wall" during endurance exercise.[14] In lieu of carbs, if you need an extra energy boost to aid your workouts during nutritional ketosis, you can use medium-chain triacylglycerols (MCT) products, such as MCT oil or MCT powder. MCTs are rapidly digested and quickly ramp up ketone levels, making them an excellent fuel to use before a ketogenic workout.

Compared to men, women naturally burn more fat and utilize fewer carbohydrates to fuel activity,[15] so the metabolic shift isn't that far off to begin with. We already have excellent fat-burning potential at our fingertips during physical activity, even before lowering carbohydrate intake. Unfortunately, most of the sports nutrition information reinforced at the gym, online, and elsewhere is geared toward men. What that means is you've likely been overreliant on carbohydrates to fuel workouts up until now. But furthermore, stop worrying that limiting carbs will somehow cancel your ability to do the physical activities you love. You can still enjoy your workouts.

Aerobic versus Anaerobic: Can You Burn Fat without Oxygen?

The intensity at which exercise is performed can affect whether carbohydrates or fat is used for fuel. During low- to moderate-intensity activity, both sugar and fat are used for fuel. During high-intensity activities, fat oxidation becomes negligible, and carbohydrates supply energy demands.[16] This energy comes from liver and muscle glycogen stores and recently ingested quick-digesting carbohydrates consumed before and during the workout.

During low- to moderate-intensity exercise, a steady supply of oxygen gets to the bloodstream, allowing aerobic metabolism to readily occur. If energy is required more rapidly than oxygen can be delivered, muscles switch to anaerobic metabolism. During exercise, this can happen when breathing becomes rapid during high-intensity activities and oxygen is limited. If you are exercising to the point where you run out of breath and gasp for air, this is anaerobic territory. At this point, the muscle's ability to burn fat is effectively switched off due to lack of oxygen, and carbohydrate fuels anaerobic metabolism.[17]

Even with restricted carbohydrate intake, your body will produce glucose via gluconeogenesis, and this can certainly help support anaerobic metabolism. But as anaerobic energy demands increase with substantial amounts of high-intensity exercise, there may be a point where low carbohydrate intake is not the most advantageous way to fuel your workout.[18] In oxygen-poor environments, our bodies can benefit from quickly digested carbohydrates to supply substrate for muscle metabolism and anaerobic energy production.

Sprinting, high-intensity interval training (HIIT), and repeated bouts of heavy weight lifting are all candidates for strategically increasing carbohydrate intake to support the workout. If these are your workouts of choice, we'll discuss implementing the diet strategies in detail in chapter 8.

Low- to moderate-intensity steady-state cardio and resistance training aren't subject to the same oxygen-restricted effects, and, therefore, fat is readily oxidized throughout the workout. A standard low-carb ketogenic intake will provide sufficient fuel during the activities; increasing carbohydrate intake for low- to moderate-intensity workouts is optional.

What Is the Best Exercise for Keto?

Just as the "best" diet is the one you stick with, the "best" exercise is one you find enjoyable and will actually show up for. I love my cardio just as much as the next gal—you'll often

Building Muscle on Keto

Like most other sport and athletic recommendations, strategies for building muscle with strength training are focused on high carbohydrate consumption.[19] I've mentioned before that many folks in bodybuilding and strength sports shun low-carb diets. Aside from the popular idea that carbs are obligatory for physical activity, the idea that low insulin impairs muscle growth and repair is a common belief working against the acceptance of low-carb diets for strength and physique. It's true that insulin works wonders for building lean body mass, and ketogenic diets lower overall insulin levels. But that doesn't mean there is no insulin response to the food we eat on a ketogenic diet; though not as dramatic a response as to carbohydrates, protein intake also elicits an insulin response, and so, too, does fat, but to a lesser extent. Low insulin does not mean *no* insulin. It is possible to gain muscle on a ketogenic diet, though low insulin levels can often be seen as a potential drawback for muscle building. To counter, you can strategically spike insulin levels with targeted carbohydrate intake around your workout, a strategy further discussed in chapter 8.

Another potential drawback of the ketogenic diet while building muscle involves the diet's hunger-suppressing effects. If you are trying to gain weight, or "bulk," you need to eat a calorie surplus, which the hunger-squashing effects of a ketogenic diet can make harder to do. If your focus involves gaining weight in an effort to build muscle, but keto makes the required calorie surplus challenging, alternating a high-carb diet for "bulking" purposes with a low-carb approach for fat loss can help you achieve your body composition goals. Remember, carbs aren't inherently bad.

Ultimately, muscle building is primarily based on protein intake.[20] During nutritional ketosis, our protein demands increase as amino acids supply the gluconeogenesis pathway. During resistance training, our muscles are broken down and then repaired during rest with an incoming flux of amino acids, which also increases protein needs. Muscle growth occurs whenever muscle protein synthesis exceeds the rate of muscle protein breakdown. The protein-sparing effects of fat adaptation can also benefit muscle growth.[21] As long as we eat adequate amounts of protein to support the demands of nutritional ketosis and exercise requirements, a keto diet can be used to build muscle. In fact, there is an entire community called Ketogains dedicated to doing this very thing—definitely check them out if this aligns with your goals.

find me in the pool doing laps for hours on end! But my time spent in the weight room is just as important, if not more so. Yet despite the documented benefits, many women avoid resistance training.[22]

We saw earlier that fat loss efforts were maximized when ketogenic diets were combined with resistance training,[23] and I've been dropping hints throughout this book that strength training is key to preserving lean body mass and attaining body composition goals. But if resistance training is so great, why do so many women avoid it?

Salvatore and Marecek[24] evaluated potential barriers for women in the weight room and found that most women reported psychosocial concerns at the root of their discomfort lifting weights.[25] Some women said that they "wouldn't want to bulk up or look too muscular," others described it as a masculine activity, and others simply didn't feel proficient with the equipment.[26] If this resonates with you at all, I see you, and I totally get it. I didn't step into a weight room until I was in my thirties! Don't let your hang-ups get in the way of self-improvement.

Resistance training can help you reduce body fat while protecting your lean body mass, it can help you build muscle to increase lean mass, and it can increase your metabolic rate.[27] If you want to lose body fat, these are all wins.

I wholeheartedly recommend resistance training for every woman. Young, old, short, tall, big, small. You don't have to compete in strongwoman competitions to benefit from lifting weights. You don't even need equipment: Pretend like you're crouching down to sit on a low bench; now stand back up. Boom. You just did a squat—and your body weight provided the resistance. It doesn't have to be complicated or scary, or even involve the weight room at the gym. And strength training will not, I repeat *will not*, make you look "bulky." It will make you look like a strong, svelte goddess. Think Jessica Biel, Halle Berry (who also does keto![28]), Eva Mendes, Gal Gadot, Angela Bassett, Alison Brie, Kate Upton—major babes. The juicy secret that all the Hollywood hardbodies seem to share is their unshakable dedication to resistance training. Every woman will benefit from resistance training, but when dieting, resistance training becomes even more critical. We want to do everything in our power to protect lean body mass, and resistance training is an effective way. For more information on female-specific weight training, check out the book *Strong Curves* by Bret Contreras.

The Female Athlete Triad: Not Properly Fueling Workouts

We briefly discussed the female athlete triad in chapter 4, but the warning not to drop calories too low is worth repeating here.

Exercise burns calories; for those involved in high levels of athletic training or who dedicate a large portion of their day to exercise, this amount of energy can be truly substantial. If you are not eating enough to meet the energy demands of your body as a result of athletic endeavors, you may be setting yourself up for menstrual disruption, decreased bone health (including osteoporosis), and eating disorders—combined, they are a medical condition known as the female athlete triad.[29] Undereating during high levels of physical activity can put you at risk for this, particularly if you are already lean, which can further disrupt hormonal balance.[30]

Keep the safe calorie deficit ranges discussed in chapter 4 in mind, and factor in your physical activity if you are performing at high levels. If you are training for a marathon and burn thousands of calories during each long run, then even a modest calorie deficit can be extreme on your body. If you are engaged in this elite level of calorie burning from physical activity alone, you don't need a calorie deficit; you need to eat. Your body needs fuel to function correctly, so give it what it needs.

So, to recap what we've learned here, you get a green light to exercise while doing the keto diet. In addition to a wide range of health benefits, working out will help you accelerate your fat loss goals when combined with a ketogenic diet. Exercise can help you burn more calories by increasing metabolic rate, preserving lean body mass, and increasing energy expenditure in your daily activities. Physical activity can also aid hormonal balance by increasing insulin sensitivity and buffering against chronically high cortisol levels.

Your physical performance may dip during the initial transition to nutritional ketosis, but once you are fat-adapted, your body will readily burn fatty acids and ketones to efficiently fuel your workouts and get back to normal. During low- to moderate-intensity workouts, you'll be able to rely purely on fat, but if you are involved in high-intensity anaerobic activities, strategic carbohydrate feedings may benefit your ability to perform.

And yes, you can even build muscle on a keto diet. Resistance training may be something you want to explore to support your fat loss and body composition goals in combination with a ketogenic diet.

Now, you've been reading a lot about *why* you should do things a certain way, but what about the *how*? Time for the fun part! The final section of this book is all about implementation.

IMPLEMENTATION OF
THE KETO DIET

Now it's time to actually *do* keto. That's right, you've made it this far, and now you are ready for the fun part: implementation! Part three of this book is all about taking action.

The dieting strategies are laid out in chapter 8 to help you choose an optimal eating pattern for your goals. You will learn about continuous carbohydrate restriction, strategic carb-ups, and when each strategy is most appropriate.

You will set up your diet in chapter 9, locking down targets and goals for your day-to-day eating.

To guide you from sugar-burner to fat-burner, chapter 10 breaks down big-picture goals and coaches you through them with incremental steps to improve your diet.

Arguably the best part about keto is all the delicious foods we get to enjoy. Chapter 11 will give you the rundown on keto-compatible foods to best meet your macronutrient goals and teach you different approaches to stay on track.

The final chapter reviews dietary sources and supplements of critical vitamins, minerals, and other compounds to keep you feeling your absolute best as you work toward your goals on keto.

Ready? Set? Go!

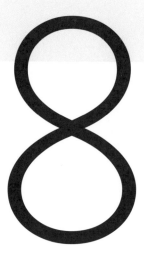

CH

8

Keto Dieting Strategies

Now it's time to dive into the juicy details of tailoring the keto diet to work for us. In this chapter, we'll review several dieting strategies that can complement the keto diet for hormonal balance, athletic performance, and body composition improvement. We'll briefly review the standard ketogenic diet and follow that with strategies to tweak the diet to best align with your goals.

Standard Keto Diet (SKD): Your Starting Point and Home Base

As we discussed in chapter 1, the conventional approach to the ketogenic diet involves restricting carbohydrates to the point where your body makes a metabolic shift to fueling itself primarily with ketones and fatty acids. By starving our body of carbohydrates, we force it to find alternative metabolic pathways to supply tissue with fuel during nutritional ketosis, and, after a period of fat adaptation, we become efficient fat-burners. During this transition, we shift our body's preferred fuel source from carbohydrate to fat.

As such, the standard ketogenic diet relies on fat as the primary fuel source. With carbohydrates out of the picture, that leaves two sources of macronutrients from which to obtain energy—protein and fat. Although protein is capable of supplying fuel for the body, it is a limited and inefficient source of energy. Fat is the primary source of energy. Protein needs are targeted, and fat supplies the remainder of the body's calorie needs. To balance energy—that is, maintain your weight—you must fill this energy void with dietary fat to provide your body with the necessary calories. However, if your goal is to lose body fat, you have access to thousands of calories of stored energy in your adipose tissue—this body fat can supply the high-fat energy requirements. To tap into this energy, you need to create a calorie deficit.

After everything you've read up to this point, you might be expecting keto to be a complex, complicated diet to figure out—*metabolic pathways*, *macronutrients*, and *energy dynamics* sound a lot more intimidating than they actually are. The truth is, implementing the standard approach to the ketogenic diet is quite straightforward. Simply keep your carb intake low (generally below 50 grams total per day), match your protein intake to your protein needs, and eat enough fat to support your goals. Voilà—you've got yourself a standard keto diet. In chapter 9, I'll walk you through determining your protein, calorie, and fat needs and goals, and in chapter 11, you will learn about the best keto food choices and different ways to keep track of your macronutrient intake.

For the most efficient path to fat-burning, the standard ketogenic diet is where I suggest everyone start. The adaptation to becoming an efficient fat-burner requires a period of low-carb dieting that usually spans several weeks. Once fat-adapted, you have the metabolic flexibility to smoothly transition back and forth between burning sugar and burning fat. This means strategically eating carbohydrates won't impede your body's fat-burning preference and capabilities, as long as you return to eating low carb in the meals, or days, following. Bypassing the period of prolonged carbohydrate restriction and jumping straight into one of the carb-based dieting strategies can lengthen the time required to become fat-adapted, so start here with the standard keto approach.

Think of the standard keto diet as your home base, where you will spend the majority of your time. It will form the basis of the other strategies, where slight tweaks will be made to suit your goals. After implementing a different approach, you will return to the standard keto way of eating until your next "deviation." Hang tough, you'll see what I mean shortly.

The long-term use of a standard ketogenic diet is most appropriate for people who have a high carbohydrate intolerance and chronic insulin resistance. For obese women, type 2 diabetics, and women with polycystic ovarian syndrome (PCOS), a standard ketogenic diet can help manage blood sugar and insulin. That's not to say this will be the ideal approach for everyone in this group forever. If at any time you wish to explore other dieting strategies,

STANDARD KETO DIET MEAL PLAN						
Sun	Mon	Tues	Wed	Thurs	Fri	Sat
SKD (<50 g carbs)	SKD (<50 g carbs)	SKD (<50 g carbs)	SKD (<50 g carbs)	SKD (<50 g carbs)	SKD (<50 g carbs)	SKD (<50 g carbs)
SKD (<50 g carbs)	SKD (<50 g carbs)	SKD (<50 g carbs)	SKD (<50 g carbs)	SKD (<50 g carbs)	SKD (<50 g carbs)	SKD (<50 g carbs)

Here's what your weekly meals will look like on a standard keto diet: pretty straightforward.

feel free to try one of the many suggestions included in this chapter. Remember, the best approach is the one that you stick with. That goes for both sides of the coin: If the standard keto approach is working for you, and you don't feel like using a carb-up strategy, by all means keep at it. I've personally used all these strategies and continue to remain flexible as my goals change. I hope you keep an open mind on your own journey and aren't afraid to experiment on your quest to better health and a better body.

Cyclical Ketogenic Diet (CKD): Routine Carb Cycling for Hormonal Balance and Performance

A cyclical keto diet is similar to a standard keto way of eating except with the introduction of carb cycling. Carb cycling consists of primarily eating a low-carbohydrate diet with planned, periodic interruptions of intentionally high-carb intake: cycles of low- and high-carb intake. Carb cycling tends to be used as an athletic strategy, but we can also incorporate intermittent carbohydrate intake to improve body composition and hormonal balance.

There is no one-size-fits-all approach to carb cycling, and your plan will depend on your individual circumstances and goals. The cyclical keto diet will be primarily based on the standard keto diet, with high-carbohydrate meals or days incorporated into your plan. If you choose to use a cyclical keto approach primarily for hormonal balance and body composition, your carb-ups will be less frequent and lower in total carbohydrate intake. For those using cyclical keto for athletic purposes, carb-ups will be more frequent and higher in overall incoming carb load.

To get the most benefit, including the metabolic flexibility afforded by fat adaptation, I recommend implementing a carb-cycling strategy after a period of low-carb dieting with the standard keto diet approach. This will give your body sufficient time to become an efficient fat-burner at rest and the ability to switch back to a fat-burning metabolism easily after a high-carb excursion.

Carb-Ups for Hormonal Balance and Low-Intensity Exercisers

1 or 2 High-Carb Meals per Week OR 1 High-Carb Refeed Day Every Two Weeks
Strategically increasing carbohydrate intake aims to address the drop in thyroid levels and rise in cortisol levels that accompany low-carb diets. While many positive hormonal changes accompany a standard keto diet, increased cortisol and decreased T3 can affect metabolic rate, affect our ability to lose body fat, and lead to large amounts of water retention.

For women already susceptible to chronically elevated cortisol and low thyroid, through various stressors or underlying hypothyroidism, these carb excursions can be particularly beneficial for rebounding thyroid and cortisol to healthy levels. Restoring balance to cortisol and thyroid function can also aid your fat loss efforts.

Menopausal and postmenopausal women using food sources of estrogen to achieve hormonal balance can also benefit from these strategic carb-ups, as the variety of phytoestrogens expands as carbohydrate restrictions are lifted.

For women not involved in high-intensity exercise, I suggest beginning carb cycling by incorporating one or two non-consecutive high-carb meals after a sufficient period of fat adaptation with standard keto. In practice, this means most of your meals will be standard keto meals, but you will plan one or two days in the week to eat a high-carb meal. The specific days you choose aren't critical, but spreading them out can help preserve the fat-burning metabolism you worked for in the initial stages of nutritional ketosis.

Realistically, you can choose to incorporate these high-carb meals more frequently than one or two times per week, but if maintaining your fat-burner metabolism is a key goal, be mindful not to let the high-carb component of your diet outweigh the low-carb one. Start with one or two high-carb meals per week, then adjust as you see fit.

Does the time of day you eat the high-carb meal matter? You can choose to eat it for breakfast, lunch, or dinner. However, there is a case to be made for holding off on carbs until later in the day. Meals high in protein and fat trigger the release of appetite-suppressing hormones and slow

Standard Keto Diet Goals

- Short-term SKD goals: A starting point—limit carbohydrates to less than 50 grams to begin the metabolic shift to nutritional ketosis.

- Interim SKD goals: Become fat adapted.

- Long-term SKD goals: Remain in a fat-burning state and use the alternative metabolic pathways to manage chronic blood sugar issues, insulin resistance, or other medically therapeutic uses. Use as a jumping-off point to other dieting strategies with strategic carb-ups.

gastric emptying rates (as discussed in chapter 6). Eating these macronutrients earlier in the day, at breakfast and lunch, can help ensure you are full and satisfied throughout the day. By the time your high-carb dinner comes around, you will be less likely to overeat. On the other hand, carbs tend to stimulate the appetite—if you start your day with carbs, managing your food intake for the remainder of the day may prove to be more challenging. Additionally, studies have shown that focusing carbohydrate intake at dinner rather than breakfast or lunch leads to decreased abdominal obesity.[1] Research also shows that consuming carbs after meat or vegetables—protein and fiber, respectively—lowers postmeal glucose and insulin patterns.[2] If you eat carbs following a day filled with protein and veggies, the smaller rise in glucose and insulin levels will be more manageable for your body.

Alternately, plan to incorporate a high-carb day every couple of weeks. In this scenario, you would eat a standard keto diet for a couple of weeks and follow up with a carb-centric day

SAMPLE CYCLICAL KETOGENIC DIET MEAL PLAN						
Sun	Mon	Tues	Wed	Thur	Fri	Sat
SKD (<50 g carbs)	SKD (<50 g carbs)	SKD (<50 g carbs)	SKD + **High-Carb Meal**	SKD (<50 g carbs)	SKD (<50 g carbs)	SKD + **High-Carb Meal**
SKD (<50 g carbs)	SKD (<50 g carbs)	SKD + **High-Carb Meal**	SKD (<50 g carbs)	SKD (<50 g carbs)	SKD + **High-Carb Meal**	SKD (<50 g carbs)

Try incorporating one or two high-carb meals per week; it will look something like this.

SAMPLE CYCLICAL KETOGENIC DIET MEAL PLAN						
Sun	Mon	Tues	Wed	Thur	Fri	Sat
SKD (<50 g carbs)	SKD (<50 g carbs)	SKD (<50 g carbs)	SKD (<50 g carbs)	SKD (<50 g carbs)	SKD (<50 g carbs)	SKD (<50 g carbs)
SKD (<50 g carbs)	SKD (<50 g carbs)	SKD (<50 g carbs)	SKD (<50 g carbs)	SKD (<50 g carbs)	SKD (<50 g carbs)	**High-Carb Day** (<25 g fat)

Or you could plan a high-carb day every two weeks, like this.

of eating. Every fourteen days or so, you temporarily switch your focus to building meals that provide adequate protein with minimal fat and meet the rest of your calorie needs with carbohydrates. Protein needs remain fixed, but you essentially swap your primary fuel source on the high-carb day. In chapter 9, we will determine your specific calorie and macronutrient needs for this dieting strategy, and in chapter 11, we will learn which high-carbohydrate foods are the best sources for carb-ups. For cyclical keto, slow-digesting carbs are preferable versus quick-digesting sources. High-carb meals and days of carb-cycling variety should be focused on whole food—complex carbohydrates rather than refined carbs. For menopausal and postmenopausal women, focus on incorporating high-carb phytoestrogens into your plan.

What to Expect After Eating High Carb?

After a brief deviation into high-carb territory, you may temporarily interrupt nutritional ketosis as your body works to burn through the sugar. With just a single high-carbohydrate meal, this will be a relatively quick shift back to ketosis and fat-burning. After an entire day of high-carb eating, expect the change to take a little longer, as your glycogen stores have filled. One way to speed the transition is by exercising with intense physical activity to burn the stored sugar. However, by simply returning to a low-carb diet, your body will bounce back to its fat-burning ways as glycogen is depleted once again.

Something else to expect after a high-carb day is a temporary increase in water weight as glycogen levels are replenished in the muscle and liver. For every gram of glycogen, there is at least three times the amount of water stored along with it.[3] As a result, this water goes straight to your muscles and can help fill out their shape; it's an aesthetically pleasing gain versus the bloated feeling of excess water retention. However, this also means you can expect your number on the scale to increase. If you have a high-carb day and suddenly your weight is up by 5 to 6 pounds (2.25 to 2.7 kg), what should you do? Relax! Remember, it's temporary, and it's just water, not body fat. It will be gone soon.

Alternately, some people describe a sudden drop in weight after eating carbohydrates following a stall in weight loss on a keto diet. The carb intake decreases the elevated stress hormone cortisol, reducing water retention. This can help explain this sudden change in weight after a high-carb intake that some dieters may experience.

Many people also complain of feeling lousy after eating high-carb meals after a period of low-carb dieting. Abdominal pain, troubles in the bathroom, and migraines are not unusual. I would argue in these cases, the quality of the carbohydrates included in the meals and underlying food sensitivities can contribute to these negative side effects of reintroducing high-carbohydrate foods, not necessarily the entire macronutrient group. The same can be seen during an elimination diet, which involves completely removing potential allergens and reintroducing them after a period of time—any negative side effects can alert you that you are sensitive, intolerant, or even allergic to that specific ingredient. If you have an underlying gluten sensitivity, you might eat a sandwich after doing keto for several months and subsequently find yourself lying curled in the fetal position cursing carbs for your pain; perhaps you should shift your focus to the content of the ingredients versus the macronutrient composition. Chances are the real culprit is a food allergen, not carbs in general. In chapter 10, we will incorporate a small-scale elimination diet to help us identify problematic ingredients, which will help you avoid planning carb-ups based on ingredients that can, potentially, hurt you and your progress.

Carb-Ups for Athletes and Frequent High-Intensity Exercisers

One or Two High-Carb Days per Week OR Targeted Keto Diet

In addition to the thyroid and cortisol rebound following high carbohydrate intake, we know glycogen storage refills. Replenishing depleted glycogen stores can be a godsend for athletes involved in high-intensity training over long durations. Recall chapter 7: Ketogenic diets are incredibly effective at burning fat for fuel during exercise, but this metabolic pathway only works efficiently in the presence of oxygen—in normal, aerobic environments. When your muscles' oxygen supply is restricted—such as when you max out your effort at the gym during high-intensity interval training, squat several hundred pounds for reps, or all-out sprint until you're a puddle lying on the floor gasping for air—then your body switches gears to an anaerobic metabolism that relies on carbs.

When glycogen levels are low, as on a ketogenic diet, the body doesn't have access to stored carbohydrates, and when oxygen is limited during high-intensity exercise, the body's fat-burning abilities become less capable. As a result, access to the body's natural energy stores is restricted. Instead, the body is left to rely on glucose produced via gluconeogenesis, using protein as an inefficient way to fuel high-intensity workouts. It's not an ideal fuel in most scenarios, but even less so at elite levels of physical activity. Without efficient fuel, performance can be impaired, and you might end up feeling really awful trying to complete your workout as planned.

The high-carbohydrate days in this plan serve to load up your body's glycogen tank. When it is unable to tap into body fat for energy during extremely high-intensity activities, you will still have the stored carbohydrate energy available to fuel the exercise.

If you are involved in high-intensity exercise, you will strategically incorporate entire high-carb days to load up glycogen storage the day before your high-intensity workout. This means your high carb days will be entirely dependent on your most intense training days.

Again, I suggest waiting to incorporate high-carb intervals until after a sufficient period of fat adaptation; however, if your athletic performance is of great concern, include the carb

SAMPLE CYCLICAL KETOGENIC DIET MEAL PLAN						
Sun	Mon	Tues	Wed	Thur	Fri	Sat
SKD (<50 g carbs)	CKD High-Carb Day (<25 g fat)	High-intensity training followed by SKD (<50 g carbs)	SKD (<50 g carbs)	CKD High-Carb Day (<25 g fat)	High-intensity training followed by SKD (<50 g carbs)	SKD (<50 g carbs)
SKD (<50 g carbs)	CKD High-Carb Day (<25 g fat)	High-intensity training followed by SKD (<50 g carbs)	SKD (<50 g carbs)	CKD High-Carb Day (<25 g fat)	High-intensity training followed by SKD (<50 g carbs)	SKD (<50 g carbs)

If you're an athlete, try a CKD plan like this one.

cycling strategy sooner. On high-intensity training days, eat a standard keto approach, and your carbs will remain low during the rest of the week as well, except for the immediate day(s) before your high-intensity workout(s).

On the day before your planned workout, swap your primary fuel source from fat to carbohydrate. We're basically reversing the macronutrient intake of the standard keto diet by limiting fat to below 25 grams (a similar amount of calories provided by 50 grams of carbs on standard keto), targeting adequate protein intake, and filling in the rest of the energy needs with slow-digesting carbs. More on this in chapters 9 and 11.

Now, this approach assumes you are not performing high-intensity training every day. If that's the case, following the guidelines to have a high-carb day before the intense training days would mean you were eating high carb every day. That's not necessarily a bad thing, but it's certainly not a keto-based diet, and the fat-adapted metabolism earned in the early phases of nutritional ketosis would soon dissipate with the continuous high carb intake. If you are doing daily high-intensity training and have your heart set on keto, consider the targeted keto diet approach discussed in the upcoming strategy section instead (see page 116).

What to Expect After a High-Carb Day Followed by High-Intensity Training?
After a day of carb-focused eating, your glycogen stores will be filled and you will have access to stored carbs for energy to use during your workout. To fuel your high-intensity exercise, your glycogen stores will be tapped and drained. The longer the physical activity, the more glycogen is depleted. Similarly, performing your workout in a fasted state can ensure glycogen is used up rather than a recent meal supplying energy. A fasting workout isn't

Is Carb Cycling Right for Everyone?

Women with impaired glucose metabolism, insulin resistance, or chronically high levels of insulin may not be the best candidates for a cyclical keto approach. The incoming carb load in these scenarios may be more detrimental if your body is unable to metabolize the nutrients effectively. Additionally, women who are severely obese may or may not have underlying insulin resistance; it would be best to stick with a standard keto approach and wait to experiment with carb cycling at a healthier weight. For women using ketogenic diets as a form of nutritional therapy and who rely on continuous ketone production to manage their symptoms, introducing carbs is not ideal and should be avoided.

Women who are athletic but perform low to moderate physical activities rather than high-intensity ones will likely not have issues with fuel accessibility or performance on a standard keto diet. For women who participate in high-intensity activities and prefer to forgo entire days of high-carb eating, we will discuss a different carb-up strategy in the next section, targeted around your workouts. If your high-intensity training activities are relatively short in duration, consider this alternative strategy, as the glycogen stores will not be fully depleted in small bouts of high-intensity training. And, finally, women who feel absolutely fantastic on a standard keto diet and aren't interested in incorporating carb-ups may be perfectly happy sticking with a standard keto approach. Consider your individual circumstances and decide what works best for you. These are not black-and-white rules to follow but guidelines and suggestions to help you tailor to your individual needs.

necessary, or even ideal for some women, but it can help speed the glycogen depletion and, essentially, bring you back to the metabolic state you were in before the high-carb day. Soon after the high-intensity glycogen-depleting workout, you will be back to fat-burning as usual.

Who Should Use the Cyclical Keto Approach?

Cyclical keto diets, or carb cycling, is most appropriate for women with low thyroid levels and chronically elevated levels of the stress hormone cortisol. Carb refeeding is also an excellent strategy for athletic women who train and compete in high-intensity sports in which performance is critical and the duration is long.

Targeted Keto Diet (TKD): Preworkout Carb Intake for Performance and Body Composition

The targeted keto diet (TKD) approach is very similar to the standard ketogenic diet; however, carbohydrates are consumed before working out (and during your workout, depending on the duration of the activity). The TKD approach is most appropriate for individuals involved in high-intensity training, to effectively fuel activities that may not provide sufficient oxygen to the muscles for fat-burning. Remember, with high-intensity activity levels, the body becomes more dependent on carbohydrates for fuel as the oxygen reaching the muscles drops and fat-burning is temporarily shut down. TDK is an alternative to the cyclical keto approach discussed in the previous section.

If you are exercising at low to moderate levels of intensity during keto, these preworkout carbohydrates aren't essential. Your body's fat-burning capabilities can handle the job. But if you're pushing your workouts to the absolute limit, eating a small amount of carbohydrates before you begin your routine can help support your efforts and performance if you choose to forgo the previous cyclical keto method. If you are trying to build muscle for strength sports, bodybuilding, or simply boosting lean mass, then these carbs serve a dual purpose by stimulating an insulin response, which promotes muscle synthesis under these circumstances.

To implement a TKD, follow the standard keto approach the majority of the time, then twenty to thirty minutes before starting your high-intensity workout, consume a quickly digested form of simple sugar. This will provide rapidly available energy in the form of carbohydrates to fuel the muscles' anaerobic metabolism as oxygen becomes limited. By the time you are done with your workout, this energy will have been used up, and you are back to standard keto, so to speak. Your fat-burning metabolism will continue and you will still reap the benefits of a keto diet, all while supporting your strenuous physical activity, strength, and/or body composition goals.

The frequency of the targeted carb intake is entirely based on the days you perform high-intensity training. If you complete intense training twice a week, your strategic carb-up will be twice a week. If daily exercise is on your agenda, daily carb-ups targeted before your workout are incorporated. The beauty of this approach is the amount of preworkout carbs is minimal, so they get entirely used up during your workout routine; ketosis and your fat-burning metabolism will go on virtually uninterrupted, aside from the time dedicated to your workout.

Begin with a targeted carb: 5 to 10 grams of carbohydrates to start (20 to 40 calories) and, if needed, up to 15 to 20 grams (60 to 80 calories). Even during carbohydrate restriction, your body will already be producing readily available glucose via gluconeogenesis—this extra preworkout intake is merely a boost to provide more efficient support. Feel free to experiment and dial in your carbs based on how you feel. To be the most effective, this small load of incoming carbs should be quickly digestible—think simple sugars. However, avoid fructose, as it goes straight to the liver rather than the muscles, making it ineffective for TKD purposes. In chapter 11, we discuss more appropriate sources of quickly digested carbs suitable for this dieting strategy.

SAMPLE TARGETED KETO DIET MEAL PLAN						
Sun	Mon	Tues	Wed	Thur	Fri	Sat
SKD (<50 g carbs)	TKD (5 to 20 g carbs 30 minutes before high-intensity workout) + SKD (<50 g carbs) throughout the rest of the day	SKD (<50 g carbs)	TKD (5 to 20 g carbs 30 minutes before high-intensity workout) + SKD (<50 g carbs) throughout the rest of the day	SKD (<50 g carbs)	TKD (5 to 20 g carbs 30 minutes before high-intensity workout) + SKD (<50 g carbs) throughout the rest of the day	SKD (<50 g carbs)
SKD (<50 g carbs)	TKD (5 to 20 g carbs 30 minutes before high-intensity workout) + SKD (<50 g carbs) throughout the rest of the day	TKD (5 to 20g carbs 30 minutes before high-intensity workout) + SKD (<50 g carbs) throughout the rest of the day	SKD (<50 g carbs)	TKD (5 to 20 g carbs 30 minutes before high-intensity workout) + SKD (<50 g carbs) throughout the rest of the day	TKD (5 to 20 g carbs 30 minutes before high-intensity workout) + SKD (<50 g carbs) throughout the rest of the day	SKD (<50 g carbs)

Here's what carbing up before workouts might look like over two weeks.

Is TKD appropriate for everyone? Not exactly. If you have an impaired response to glucose, insulin resistance, or metabolic issues that require a continued state of ketosis, it may be best to avoid a concentrated carb-up before you hit the gym. With low- to moderate-intensity workouts, a keto-adapted body will be able to fuel the activity sufficiently. It goes without saying, but I'll say it anyway: There is no need to consume quick-digesting carbohydrates if you aren't working out. If you are interested in an alternative keto diet strategy that includes carbs without an obligatory exercise component, you may benefit from carb cycling with complex carbs, as previously described in the cyclical keto diet strategy section (see page 110). Or perhaps eating in a way that coincides with your hormonal cycle is an appropriate fit, as discussed in the next section (see page 119). Also, if a standard keto diet feels like it is working for you and supporting your high-intensity workouts, don't feel obligated to add preworkout carbs just because it's an option. This is your journey; you're in charge. Listen to your body and do what feels right.

Luteal Keto Diet (LKD): Eating for Your Hormonal Cycle

As we learned in chapter 5, shifts in estrogen and progesterone levels throughout the month affect our metabolic rate and eating habits. The hormonal fluctuations also affect our inherent ability to metabolize carbohydrates. In the first portion of the cycle, we are most sensitive to the effects of insulin, and we lose this sensitivity in the latter part of the cycle. Syncing our macronutrient strategy with our body's natural ability to effectively burn carbs—or not—can give us an edge when it comes to achieving both our body composition goals and hormonal balance. The luteal keto strategy is based on focusing carb intake or carb cycling efforts in the first part of our hormonal cycle while minimizing carb intake in the second portion to help optimize our efforts. If you were wondering why I strongly suggested tracking your period, here's the reason.

Sticking to a standard keto diet during the luteal phase can counteract the adverse effects that accompany the second portion of the hormonal cycle. The progesterone-driven luteal phase of the menstrual cycle is riddled with insulin resistance, an aggressive increase in hunger and appetite, intense cravings, a drop in the thermic effect of food, and impulsive decision making. As a result, overeating is a huge issue for many women during the final weeks of their cycle. Hundreds of extra calories consumed each day can quickly become thousands of excess calories during one cycle. Without an effective way to manage this, you could be packing on body fat every four weeks like clockwork.

The appetite-suppressing effects of the keto diet address the increased drive to eat and annihilate cravings. Without the nagging cravings and explosive hunger, we are also less likely to engage in the impulsive eating characteristic of this time. Ensuring adequate protein is consumed with well-balanced keto macros can provide an increase in the thermic effect of food. And, of course, a standard keto diet can bypass insulin resistance by offering an alternative metabolic pathway. By keeping our carbohydrate intake low during the luteal phase, we can skirt the effects of insulin resistance and prevent ourselves from overeating and gaining body fat as a result. Imagine if each luteal phase was spent burning body fat instead of gaining it!

On the flip side of the luteal phase, we have the estrogen-driven follicular phase, the first portion of the hormonal cycle. As estrogen rises as the dominant hormone, our metabolic rate drops slightly, but sensitivity to insulin increases. This is the time our bodies naturally increase their ability to metabolize carbs. If there were ever a time to increase carbohydrate consumption, the follicular phase undoubtedly makes the most sense.

To remain fat-adapted, we must ensure the majority of our dietary intake is low carb rather than high carb. Knowing our ability to process carbs is higher during the initial phase of the cycle, we can reason that carb cycling during this time is actually more effective than during the last portion of the cycle. Rather than sticking to one of the previously discussed schedules for strategic carb-ups continually, consider limiting their use to the follicular phase of the menstrual cycle or lowering the total amount of carbs used for carb-ups during the luteal phase.

To optimize your body's natural rhythms and support your goals, eat a standard keto diet during the luteal phase. It can help alleviate cravings, hunger, and decreased insulin sensitivity. While carb cycling during the follicular phase when the body is most insulin sensitive, we can reset cortisol and thyroid levels, fuel intense workouts, and even work to develop lean mass.

This could be implemented in a variety of ways. Perhaps you schedule a high-carb day to align with when your period starts, marking the beginning of your follicular phase and hormonal cycle. Or maybe you enjoy a high-carb meal on the first day of your menstrual bleed, followed by one or two high-carb meals per week until ovulation. For those involved in ongoing high-intensity training, this could also mean implementing a cyclical keto approach of high-carb days before activity during the follicular phase followed by a targeted keto approach on training days during the luteal phase. Or during the luteal

SAMPLE LUTEAL KETO DIET MEAL PLAN							
Phase	Sun	Mon	Tues	Wed	Thur	Fri	Sat
Follicular	1st day of period						
SKD + **High-Carb Meal**	SKD (<50 g carbs)	SKD (<50 g carbs)	SKD + **High-Carb Meal**	SKD (<50 g carbs)	SKD (<50 g carbs)	SKD + **High-Carb Meal**	SKD (<50 g carbs)
Follicular	SKD (<50 g carbs)	SKD (<50 g carbs)	SKD + **High-Carb Meal**	SKD (<50 g carbs)	SKD (<50 g carbs)	SKD + **High-Carb Meal**	SKD (<50 g carbs)
Luteal	Ovulation						
SKD (<50 g carbs)	SKD (<50 g carbs)	SKD (<50 g carbs)	SKD (<50 g carbs)	SKD (<50 g carbs)	SKD (<50 g carbs)	SKD (<50 g carbs)	SKD (<50 g carbs)
Luteal	SKD (<50 g carbs)	SKD (<50 g carbs)	SKD (<50 g carbs)	SKD (<50 g carbs)	SKD (<50 g carbs)	SKD (<50 g carbs)	SKD (<50 g carbs)

Here's a sample schedule for optimizing hormonal balance.

SAMPLE LUTEAL KETO DIET MEAL PLAN							
Phase	Sun	Mon	Tues	Wed	Thur	Fri	Sat
Follicular	*1st day of period*						
SKD (<50 g carbs)	**CKD High-Carb Day** (<25 g fat)	High-Intensity Training followed by SKD (<50 g carbs)	SKD (<50 g carbs)	**CKD High-Carb Day** (<25 g fat)	High-Intensity Training followed by SKD (<50 g carbs)	SKD (<50 g carbs)	SKD (<50 g carbs)
Follicular	SKD (<50 g carbs)	**CKD High-Carb Day** (<25 g fat)	High-Intensity Training followed by SKD (<50 g carbs)	SKD (<50 g carbs)	**CKD High-Carb Day** (<25 g fat)	High-Intensity Training followed by SKD (<50 g carbs)	SKD (<50 g carbs)
Luteal	*Ovulation*						
SKD (<50 g carbs)	TKD (5 to 20 g carbs 30 minutes before high-intensity workout) + SKD (<50 g carbs) throughout the rest of the day	SKD (<50 g carbs)	TKD (5 to 20 g carbs 30 minutes before high-intensity workout) + SKD (<50 g carbs) throughout the rest of the day	SKD (<50 g carbs)	TKD (5 to 20 g carbs 30 minutes before high-intensity workout) + SKD (<50 g carbs) throughout the rest of the day	SKD (<50 g carbs)	SKD (<50 g carbs)
Luteal	SKD (<50 g carbs)	TKD (5 to 20 g carbs 30 minutes before high-intensity workout) + SKD (<50 g carbs) throughout the rest of the day	SKD (<50 g carbs)	TKD (5 to 20 g carbs 30 minutes before high-intensity workout) + SKD (<50 g carbs) throughout the rest of the day	SKD (<50 g carbs)	TKD (5 to 20 g carbs 30 minutes before high-intensity workout) + SKD (<50 g carbs) throughout the rest of the day	SKD (<50 g carbs)

This example schedule is for high-intensity athletes.

SAMPLE LUTEAL KETO DIET MEAL PLAN							
Phase	Sun	Mon	Tues	Wed	Thur	Fri	Sat
Follicular	1st day of period						
High-Carb Day (<25 g fat)	High-Carb Day (<25 g fat)	High-Carb Day (<25 g fat)	High-Carb Day (<25 g fat)	High-Carb Day (<25 g fat)	High-Carb Day (<25 g fat)	High-Carb Day (<25 g fat)	High-Carb Day (<25 g fat)
Follicular	High-Carb Day (<25 g fat)	High-Carb Day (<25 g fat)	High-Carb Day (<25 g fat)	High-Carb Day (<25 g fat)	High-Carb Day (<25 g fat)	High-Carb Day (<25 g fat)	High-Carb Day (<25 g fat)
Luteal	Ovulation						
SKD (<50 g carbs)	SKD (<50 g carbs)	SKD (<50 g carbs)	SKD (<50 g carbs)	SKD (<50 g carbs)	SKD (<50 g carbs)	SKD (<50 g carbs)	SKD (<50 g carbs)
Luteal	SKD (<50 g carbs)	SKD (<50 g carbs)	SKD (<50 g carbs)	SKD (<50 g carbs)	SKD (<50 g carbs)	SKD (<50 g carbs)	SKD (<50 g carbs)

Here's an example of using keto only during the luteal phase.

Who Is the Luteal Keto Approach *Not* For?

This hormonal cycle approach to keto isn't particularly useful for women who no longer have menstrual cycles. That's not to say those alternating periods of carb cycling with strict low-carbohydrate intake won't have benefits, but the underlying hormonal shifts that provide structure for optimizing nutrient intake will be absent. For women who are postmenopausal or experiencing other menstrual interruptions, using any one of the other dieting strategies discussed may be more appropriate.

Additionally, this strategy is largely based on the concept that insulin resistance decreases in the follicular phase. However, there are plenty of women who are continuously insulin resistant, all the time, regardless of menstrual phase. For women who fall into the unabated insulin resistance category, the standard keto approach may provide the most benefit.

phase, a standard keto approach may be the most ideal. Ultimately, it's up to you how best to incorporate this method, and it's dependent on your own unique hormonal cycle. Bear in mind, the examples on the preceding pages are more for helping you visualize the possibilities rather than strict schedules and rules to follow.

However you choose to apply this strategy, remember your body is more responsive to carbs during the time between your menstrual bleed and ovulation, while carbs are less agreeable in the time following ovulation up until the first day of your menstrual bleed. In the follicular phase, i.e., preovulation, carbohydrates can be strategic. In the luteal phase, i.e., postovulation, carbohydrates can work against your fat loss goals.

Alternately, we can entertain the idea of eating a high-carb diet during the follicular phase and a low-carb keto diet during the luteal phase. While this approach is not necessarily conducive to fat adaptation, it aligns with the body's inherent ability to properly metabolize and counteract the adverse effects on body composition and fat loss efforts often seen during the luteal phase.

Who Is This "Luteal Keto" Approach Most Appropriate For?

The women who will benefit from this approach the most are those willing and able to track their menstrual cycles. If you have a period, I highly recommend tracking it for insight into your hormonal balance and optimizing your diet strategy. Naturally, there will be women who are not interested in monitoring start to finish, but that telltale first day of your menstrual bleed is hard to ignore. Even without an official tracking method, you can use that initial sign as a cue that carb cycling or increased carb intake is going to be most effective during this time.

Breaking Up with Your Diet: Planned Diet Breaks

When people talk about eating outside their planned diet regimen, the language they use makes it sound as if they committed an unethical act—they "cheated," they "fell off the wagon," they "failed." But thinking back to the food-as-fuel analogy, would you beat yourself up if you put too much gas in your car? Of course not!

Considering that I'm writing this book, this might come as a surprise: I absolutely *hate* diets! The mind-set that tends to come with the territory can be extremely unforgiving. People start to associate being on a diet as "good" and off a diet as "bad." Even worse, many diets prescribe such strict protocols to follow that it sends the message that a minor deviation from the rules is a punishable crime. Keto dieters are not immune to this phenomenon: Ketosis is "good," while being out of ketosis is "bad"; carrots, bell peppers, and beets have carbs, so they must be avoided at all costs (as an aside, these veggies never made anyone fat—please stop blaming them); any amount of sugar put into your body is "toxic" or "poison."

I will be the first to admit I have picked out carrots that came in my salads, read the word "sugar" deep in the ingredients list on a nutrition label and recoiled in horror, stressed and obsessed about the "rules" of keto, meticulously tracked every morsel, and wallowed in a sad pool of grief, guilt, and self-loathing after eating "too many" carbs. This isn't healthy living. These are the bright red flags of disordered eating. One reason I was so excited to write this book was to share the many mistakes I have personally made, so you don't make them, too; this is right up there at the top of my Don't Do What I Did list!

Keeping an open mind and flexible attitude can certainly help when venturing into carb cycling or incorporating strategic carb-ups, which are decidedly *not* standard keto practice. Taking this one step further, allowing more flexibility into your diet mind-set can help you bounce back when things don't go as planned or expected.

Throughout this book, I've continued to emphasize that carbs are not quintessentially evil, and not all carbs are the same. I don't want you to develop an unhealthy relationship with your food, think of any given nutrient as an enemy, or consider a diet as a partner you must remain faithful to. Instead, I much rather that you develop a positive, healthy, open relationship with your food and simply use keto dieting as a tool or strategy to meet your goals, not a measure of self-worth. An all-or-nothing mind-set doesn't serve you well when it comes to nourishing your body. Period.

I encourage you to consider taking a break from your diet if you start feeling like you're approaching "I am a failure because I ate ___" territory. Even if you don't experience these negative feelings (yay!), planning a diet break can be helpful for long-term compliance, hormonal balance, and even body composition. The increased carbs will serve to boost your thyroid, put elevated cortisol to rest, and provide optimal insulin levels for building lean mass.

Plain and simple, a keto diet break offers yet another strategy. Follow keto for a period to be used for effective fat loss, then plan a break. A break means no carb restrictions, calorie restrictions, or any other restrictions not directly related to medical needs or allergies. Eat *ad libitum* with foods of your choice.

Continuous energy restriction can induce physiological effects that hinder further weight loss. Remember, your body is doing a lot of sneaky things to fight back against calorie restriction and doing what it can to hold on to stored energy. Deliberately taking a break to eat at maintenance calories for a time can help alleviate the adaptive responses to energy restriction and thereby *increase* the efficiency of weight loss.[4]

This isn't intended to be a free-for-all or excuse to binge-eat but a time to reset your body's adaptations to prevent weight loss, revitalize your mind-set, and prevent feelings of deprivation. Maybe you're going on vacation and a diet break to enjoy the local food is

Continuous energy restriction can induce physiological effects that hinder further weight loss.

well warranted. Perhaps doing keto over the holidays proves to be particularly challenging with family, friends, and coworkers rejoicing around traditional foods. As the saying goes, "It's not what you eat between Christmas and New Year's; it's what you eat between New Year's and Christmas."

If you are concerned about losing progress during a break from keto, I suggest doing what many bodybuilders do in the off-season: bulk. If you are eating a higher-carbohydrate diet, use that to your advantage and get some resistance training in. Not in a punishing, compensatory way to burn calories but as a long-term strategy to improve your metabolic rate and body composition. As long as you continue eating adequate protein, this period can be used to your advantage to build lean mass more efficiently using the anabolic effects of insulin and increased calorie intake when combined with resistance training.[5] During this time, you may gain a small amount of weight as muscle increases, but you will be decreasing your overall body fat percentage.

If you continue to eat maintenance-level calories during this time rather than a surplus or deficit, you can slowly lose fat while gaining muscle and strength. For those at or near their goal weight, this can be an effective way to change body composition without "dieting" per se. As you get leaner, you will continue to lose volume and drop dress sizes, even though the number on the scale will stay relatively static. After all, muscle is denser than body fat. For those who have chosen to use keto to shed body fat effectively, but don't view it as a long-term solution or way of eating, I highly recommend considering this option when you officially break up with your diet.

If you still have a reasonable amount of fat to lose, you can return to keto with your recently increased metabolic rate and *improved* body composition. If you wish to continue with keto as a long-term strategy for its myriad health benefits even after you've reached your goal weight, remember to increase your calorie intake to align with your new goal: maintaining your progress. The choice is yours, and yours alone. Long story short, it's definitely okay to take breaks.

In summary, there are a variety of ways to implement keto, even if the methods don't necessarily involve the traditional approach to the diet. Carb cycling, targeted carb-ups, and menstrual cues can all provide alternative strategies to reach your goals and make the diet work best for you. Additionally, planned diet breaks away from keto can provide physiological and psychological mind-set benefits.

Next up, we learn how to set up calorie and macronutrient needs based on the dieting strategies described in this chapter.

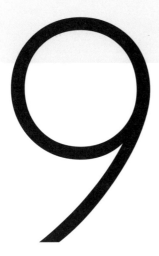

Setting Up the Diet: How Much Should You Eat?

In the last chapter, we reviewed the various keto-based dieting strategies. By now you have a pretty good idea of which method is the best fit for you in the beginning and where you foresee taking your diet in the long run.

In this chapter, we are going to establish the foundational structure of your diet by setting your macronutrient goals. Essentially, we'll figure out how much you should eat and determine the macronutrient breakdown—the amount of protein, carbs, and fats that best supports your goals. This ensures you eat an appropriate amount of each macronutrient to lose body fat, preserve lean body mass, and remain in nutritional ketosis.

To do this, you need to determine:

1. Your energy needs by calculating your TDEE and appropriate calorie deficit
2. Your protein needs based on lean body mass

3. Appropriate carb levels based on dieting strategy

4. Fat levels based on body composition goals and dieting strategy.

The equations found in this chapter aren't meant to scare you off but to provide background information. Rest assured, math is *not* required to do keto. These values are simply intended to provide you with a working knowledge of calorie needs to maintain or lose weight with macronutrient goals geared toward nutritional ketosis, preservation of lean body mass, and, of course, how strategic carb increases affect overall intake.

You will notice that once calorie needs are determined for each macronutrient, the value is subsequently converted to grams. At first, this may seem like an extra step, but it's to help you in the long run. Nutrition information listed on labels and in databases is all listed in grams. Chapter 11 will help you connect the dots between the food you eat and the nutrient values determined here.

Keto Calculator for Women

Here's a shortcut tool designed to do the math and assist you with dieting strategy details. The calculator tool on my website has been designed specifically to align with this book; it takes into account fat loss and diet strategies, and, most importantly, it's just for women. It's a huge time saver and streamlines the entire process laid out in the following pages. The keto calculator can be found at ketogasm.com/keto-calculator.

Keto calculators are a popular tool for people just beginning the diet. They help align energy needs with keto macronutrient goals to provide a basic structure to meet your big-picture nutritional needs. There are hundreds of keto-based calculator options on the web, though not all are created with the same context and goals in mind. The formulas and underlying frames of reference differ from tool to tool, and, as a result, the outcomes vary wildly. Just as there are many *reasons* to do keto, there are a variety of *ways* to do keto. Many calculators base macronutrient suggestions and calculations on ratios useful for ketone therapy (as discussed in chapter 1) rather than optimal fat loss purposes. And while there are currently several excellent options that deliver appropriate macros for fat loss, they are structured for use with a standard keto diet only. Thus, a little manual tweaking would be required to accommodate any one of our alternative diet strategies. Finally, to my knowledge, no other online tool has been developed exclusively for women. I recommend using this book's supplemental calculator for a relevant and convenient transition.

Side note: if you have a male keto-dieting buddy, do them a favor and tell them about the Ketogains macro calculator for men. This is the tool I have recommended for years to any guy beginning a standard keto diet.

Determining Your Energy Needs

To figure out what your body needs in terms of energy, we'll start with what you normally expend—total daily energy expenditure. Then we'll figure out what you'll need to take in to meet your goals.

Total Daily Energy Expenditure

The first thing we need to do is determine our body's energy needs, also known as our total daily energy expenditure (TDEE). Think back to chapter 4—this is the value that tallies all the factors contributing to "calories out," or what our body is spending to fuel our metabolic rate, activities, and thermic effect of food. TDEE will provide the foundation for how our keto macronutrient goals are partitioned. Remember: Macronutrients *are* calories; we just need to set them up in a way to support nutritional ketosis, fat loss, and preservation of lean mass.

As I've said before (page 127), there are a variety of formulas that can be used to determine TDEE and even more online tools available to perform the calculations. The values can differ from equation to equation; after all, these are simply mathematical models used to make predictions, not an exact science. Right out of the gate, we are dealing with ballpark estimates, so if you are a diet perfectionist who obsesses over exacting numbers, take a deep breath and exhale your meticulous attention to detail. Most formulas and even nutrition data on labels and databases are intended to be reasonably accurate, not precise. Let go of laser-like precision when it comes to your diet, because it doesn't really exist. Reasonably accurate is good enough.

If you use the calculator on Ketogasm, TDEE calories will compute automatically based on your input and provide the basis for the remaining values. This supplemental tool uses the Mifflin–St. Jeor equation for women to determine the resting metabolic rate (RMR). This formula was developed to improve the accuracy of RMR measurements in people with excess body fat using a range of individuals from healthy weight to severely obese. When compared to other RMR formulas, the Mifflin–St. Jeor formula showed the lowest bias and was the most accurate formula in both normal-weight and overweight females.[1] In other words, this is the most reasonably accurate formula we can use for resting metabolic rate within our context.

The calculations are a little complicated, and naturally, I don't expect you to perform them manually. I recommend using a TDEE calculator to really speed the diet setup along.

Determining Your Calorie Defcit

This TDEE value is going to represent the number of calories you need to eat to maintain energy balance. If your TDEE is 2,000 calories, you will eat 2,000 calories to keep your weight stable—pretty straightforward. If your goal is to lose weight, then we have to subtract some of the incoming calories to create the calorie deficit we've discussed. In chapter 4, I laid out a table to illustrate safe calorie deficits. A deficit doesn't need to be a dramatic

Maintenance Keto Macros

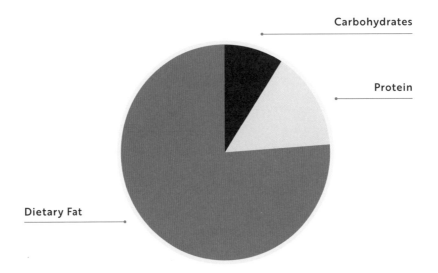

Carbohydrates

Protein

Dietary Fat

Keto Fat Loss Macros

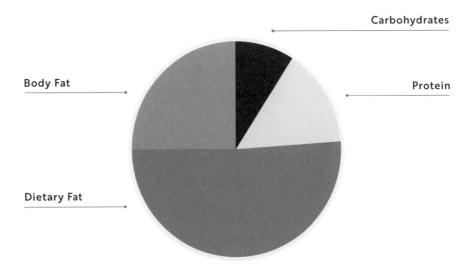

Carbohydrates

Protein

Body Fat

Dietary Fat

slash in calories; if you are concerned about your hormonal balance and lean body mass, it most definitely shouldn't! Going beyond a 25 percent calorie deficit risks loss of lean mass, menstrual interruptions, and further driving thyroid levels down and cortisol up.

Women who have more body fat to lose are generally able safely to maintain higher levels of calorie restriction without losing lean mass or throwing their hormones out of whack. But leaner women need to take a more conservative approach to support hormonal balance and lean body mass.

For women above a healthy weight, aim for a max 20 to 25 percent calorie deficit. For women at a healthy weight interested in becoming leaner, don't go beyond a 15 to 20 percent deficit, or eat at maintenance calories and implement resistance training as discussed in the previous chapter (see page 100).

Let's pretend we have a woman named Molly who is above a healthy weight, and her TDEE is around 2,700 calories per day. Molly would be an excellent candidate to eat at the higher range of our safe, moderate calorie deficits while she's on the keto diet. If she has a really high body fat percentage, then an even steeper deficit may be appropriate for short periods. However, even with high body fat, extreme deficits are not sustainable long term. Your body fights against severe energy restriction through various hormonal responses and signals, and efforts can prove to be futile. Using the highest end of our safe calorie range, we can see what this might look like in practice.

> 2,700 TDEE × 25 percent calorie deficit = 675-calorie deficit
> TDEE − calorie deficit = how many calories to eat in a day to lose body fat
> 2,700 TDEE − 675-calorie deficit = 2,025 calories to eat in a day to lose body fat

By eating 2,025 calories per day, Molly is at a 675-calorie deficit each day and a 4,725-calorie deficit per week. As she loses weight, her energy needs and TDEE will also decrease. As such, I recommend reassessing TDEE and adjusting incoming calorie levels after significant weight loss—every 5 to 10 pounds, depending on how much weight you actually have to lose.

How many calories you eat in a day will also determine your keto macronutrients, which we will take a look at in the upcoming protein, carbs, and fat sections.

Continuous Calorie Restriction versus Calorie Cycling

Molly's example illustrates a continuous daily calorie deficit. But the truth is you don't need to be in a calorie deficit every single day to lose weight. Rather, you need an overall deficit, and that can be achieved just as effectively with intermittent calorie restriction. Your cumulative efforts are more meaningful than what happens over the course of one day. Just as we discussed the use of carb cycling in the previous chapter, I want to introduce the concept of calorie cycling as we discuss energy needs.

EXAMPLE CONTINUOUS CALORIE RESTRICTION PLAN							
Sun	Mon	Tues	Wed	Thur	Fri	Sat	Totals
Eat: 2,025 calories	Eat: 2,025 calories	Eat: 2,025 calories	Eat: 2,025 calories	Eat: 2,025 calories	Eat: 2,025 calories	Eat: 2,025 calories	Calories Consumed: **14,175**
Daily Deficit: 675 calories	Daily Deficit: 675 calories	Daily Deficit: 675 calories	Daily Deficit: 675 calories	Daily Deficit: 675 calories	Daily Deficit: 675 calories	Daily Deficit: 675 calories	Weekly Deficit: **4,725 calories**

Here's what Molly's meal plan might look like with her 2,700-calorie TDEE and a 25 percent calorie deficit.

As an alternative to restricting calories daily, we can choose to restrict on certain days and bounce back to maintenance levels on others. To accommodate the higher-calorie days, the reduced-calorie days will be a fair bit lower than if you were to eat at a continuous deficit. However, the overall deficit achieved remains the same.

Preceding, Molly restricted calories daily at a 25 percent deficit to achieve a total deficit of 4,725 calories for the week. If she introduced calorie cycling, she could achieve the same deficit in a variety of ways. Maybe she finds it easier to maintain a calorie deficit during the workweek, but during the weekend she has difficulty sticking to her planned deficit because she loves to cook and that's her time to try new recipes. What if the calorie restriction is lifted over the weekend and those two days are spent balanced with her daily TDEE, while Monday through Friday she further reduces the calories? Turn the page to see what that would look like.

Even though she ate maintenance level calories two days, she still ended up with an identical outcome for the week simply by adjusting her calorie-restricted days.

The possible calorie cycling patterns are truly endless. My mentioning calorie cycling isn't intended to complicate things, but to show a viable alternative to continuous calorie restriction in the event it is something you find yourself struggling with. If you know certain days of

EXAMPLE OF WEEKEND CALORIE CYCLING							
Sun	Mon	Tues	Wed	Thur	Fri	Sat	Totals
Eat: 2,700 calories	Eat: 1,755 calories	Eat: 1,755 calories	Eat: 1,755 calories	Eat: 1,755 calories	Eat: 1,755 calories	Eat: 2,700 calories	Calories Consumed: **14,175**
Daily Deficit: 0 calories	Daily Deficit: 945 calories	Daily Deficit: 945 calories	Daily Deficit: 945 calories	Daily Deficit: 945 calories	Daily Deficit: 945 calories	Daily Deficit: 0 calories	Weekly Deficit: **4,725 calories**

This sample assumes a 2,700-calorie TDEE and a 25 percent overall calorie deficit.

the week consistently present diet and calorie restriction obstacles, consider calorie cycling to counter that. It's certainly not necessary, but it's an option that *any* keto dieting strategy can make use of.

To be clear, you don't necessarily have to plan, calculate, and juggle where the calories fall. Calorie cycling can be a more intuitive process. There may be some days you barely feel like eating and other days you are surprisingly hungry; keto has amazing appetite-suppressing effects, but that doesn't mean you will be immune to days when you feel like eating everything in sight. It definitely happens. Allow yourself to eat more on the days you have a healthy appetite and less on days where you don't really feel like it. Crunching numbers doesn't need to be a part of your game plan for you to benefit from this process.

Calorie cycling has its benefits as well, similar to those of diet breaks discussed in the previous chapter but on a more regular basis. When calories are increased, it signals to the body that access to food is not limited, and the body's physiologic adaptations to prevent weight loss are put to rest.[4] Additionally, intermittent calorie restriction may be more effective at reducing abdominal fat than daily calorie restriction[5]—a win for improved body composition!

How many meals a day should you eat? Honestly, that's your call. Much like the dieting strategies, how you choose to fuel your body is completely in your hands—and that includes how frequently you eat. Whether you feel like eating three squares, five to six little meals, or saving it all up for one big feast, have at it. Just be sure you eat enough—don't let your eating patterns and meal frequency cause a dangerous calorie deficit or prevent you from getting adequate nutrition. You need to get enough protein, vitamins, minerals, and energy if you want to improve your health and body composition rather than run it into the ground. I don't believe in imposing windows of time when it is and isn't "okay to eat." Although tools such as intermittent fasting can most definitely help provide structure and improve compliance for some, I feel calorie restriction can be accomplished naturally without designating a set time frame to allow your body nourishment. Sometimes simply listening to your body is the best compass.

Protein Is Queen

Now that we know your TDEE, we need to figure out your body's protein needs. We are going to set this macro first because it is absolutely critical regardless of where you fall on the diet spectrum: low carb, high carb, vegan, carnivore, you name it—you need protein. After all, proteins are the body's building blocks. Protein is essential for a plethora of biological functions, including hormone production, but when it comes to dieting and weight loss, adequate protein intake is a primary requirement for maintaining lean body mass.

The good news is your protein needs remain relatively static as long as your lean mass stays the same. Chances are you probably already eat enough protein. I've been harping on the importance of eating adequate amounts of protein this entire book, but not necessarily to get you to consume *more*. Instead, I want to encourage you to continue eating enough protein. Unfortunately, many people start keto and significantly drop their protein intake, based on some myths, misconceptions, and misunderstandings discussed in previous chapters.

Let's set the record straight. If you are a woman using keto for fat loss and hormonal balance—*not* ketone therapy—there is no need to intentionally limit or restrict protein intake for the sake of ketone production. Cutting protein intake to lose weight faster does not improve body composition; it causes muscle loss instead of body fat loss and massively decreases your metabolism. Although eating "too much" protein does not provide any inherent benefits, there is little evidence that protein overfeeding causes adverse effects in the general population.[6]

So how much protein is adequate for a keto diet? Between 0.6 and 1 gram per pound (454 g) of lean body mass.[7]

Anything within this range is a reasonable goal, though protein needs do increase with physical activity. If you are involved in any form of exercise, target the higher end of the range for best results.

Because we are basing protein needs on lean body mass, we need to figure out how much lean mass you have. There are a variety of methods to determine body composition, and we discussed them in chapter 4 while exploring body fat measurements. A DEXA scan is the gold standard for this purpose, and if you are interested in getting a professional assessment, I highly recommend it. There are other machines and physical tools that can measure your body fat, too. Once you know how much body fat you carry, you can easily calculate your lean body mass.

Lean body mass = body weight − fat mass

The most cost-effective (free!) way to get an estimate of lean body mass is using a calculator. The U.S. Navy body composition formula for women is recommended as it has been found to be more reliable for women than other body fat prediction formulas.[8] You will need a fabric measuring tape to measure your neck, natural waist, and hips on bare skin. Measure in centimeters. One good calculator can be found at www.calculator.net/body-fat-calculator.html.

Once you have your body fat percentage, you can determine your fat mass. Then, subtract the fat mass from the total body weight to determine your lean body mass.

Now let's imagine a woman named Sherry who is trying to figure out her lean body mass. She weighs 200 pounds, she stands 5 feet 4 inches (1.6 m) tall, her neck is 15 inches (38 cm), her waist is 38 inches (96.5 cm), and her hips are 50 inches (127 cm).

Her body fat percentage using the U.S. Navy method is 49.8 percent, so her body fat weighs 99.6 pounds (45 kg):

200 pounds (90.7 kg) × 49.8 percent body fat = 99.6 pounds (45 kg) fat mass

That means Sherry has 100.4 pounds (45.5 kg) lean body mass:

200 pounds (90.7 kg) − 99.6 pounds (45 kg) fat mass =
100.4 pounds (45.5 kg) of lean body mass

Now that Sherry knows her lean body mass, she understands she needs to eat adequate protein to protect it, especially as she's dieting. Using the protein range of 0.6 to 1.0 grams of protein per pound (454 g) of lean body mass, Sherry can determine appropriate protein levels for her body.

Minimun: (0.6 g protein ÷ lb lean body mass) × 100.4 pounds LBM =
60.24 grams of protein per day

Maximum: (1 g protein ÷ lb lean body mass) × 100.4 pounds LBM =
100.4 grams of protein per day

Adequate daily protein: 60 to 100 grams of protein per day

Sherry needs to aim for a bare minimum intake of 60 grams of protein per day but is well within her range up to 100 grams in a day. If Sherry remains active, she will likely do fine

Protein Goals for All Dieting Strategies

Aim to get 0.6 to 1.0 gram of protein per pound (454 g) of lean body mass.

in the lower end of the spectrum, but if she adds workouts to her routine, it would be in her best interest to aim for the higher end.

For most women who aren't physically active, I recommend purposefully targeting the middle of the adequate protein range, or 0.8 gram per pound (454 g) of lean mass. This will keep you securely in the zone of protecting your lean body mass while allowing you to enjoy the benefits of slightly higher protein intake mentioned throughout the book. Remember, it's not "high protein"; it's adequate protein.

Carbs: Limit or Leverage?

Of all the macronutrients, carbohydrates are the only nonessential ones. That's because the body has its own mechanism for producing carbohydrates as needed when dietary carb intake is low.

For a standard keto diet and during the initial periods of fat adaptation, we will need to intentionally limit our carbohydrate intake to induce nutritional ketosis. Though remaining on a standard keto diet is an entirely viable option for many women, particularly those who are battling insulin resistance and other forms of impaired glucose metabolism, long-term carbohydrate restriction has the potential to bring about negative hormonal shifts, specifically decreased thyroid function and increased cortisol levels that drive down our metabolic rate and negatively affect our ability to lose weight. And during some forms of high-intensity exercise, it's difficult for the body's internal glucose production to keep up with the increased demands of anaerobic exercise. When limited carbs are interfering with your goals, carbohydrates can be used as leverage to trigger the hormones to bounce back, fight through a weight loss stall, and efficiently fuel intense workouts.

Carbs on a Standard Keto Diet (SKD)

Throughout this book, limiting carbohydrates to fewer than 50 grams has been my default value for achieving nutritional ketosis and maintaining a standard keto diet. In practice, this number will fluctuate dependent on individual carbohydrate tolerance and personal preference, but 50 grams is a reasonable limit for most.

But we've also learned not all carbohydrates are created equal. We are interested in unprocessed, unrefined, slow-digesting, fibrous sources of carbohydrates for most standard keto needs. We'll discuss specific sources that deliver these carbohydrates in chapter 11, but bringing it up here allows me to introduce the concept of "net" carbs. Net carbs are total carbohydrate minus fiber.

Net carbs = total carbs − dietary fiber

The net carb concept revolves around the idea that not all carbs "count," per se. Fiber is largely undigested by humans, mainly traveling through the digestive tract as roughage provided by plant cell walls. So, subtracting dietary fiber–based carbs from the total carb count provides the number of carbs that do "count"—those that affect glucose metabolism and nutritional ketosis. It's more of a mind-set thing, but in subtracting the fiber from your food, you arrive at an artificially "lower" carb count, or "net" carbs. When eating ideal carb sources, there is no difference between 50 grams of total carbs versus 25 grams of fiber and 25 grams of net carbs. If someone tells you they are doing keto and eating 20 to 30 grams of net carbs per day, chances are their total carbohydrate intake is closer to 50 grams per day, unless they are restricting even vegetables.

Carb Goals for Standard Keto Diet (SKD)

- Total carb intake:
  Up to 50 grams daily

- Dietary fiber intake:
  Target 25 grams daily

- Net carb intake:
  Up to 20 to 30 grams daily

Fiber is proven to be useful in the prevention and management of many diseases. It also has antioxidant properties, improves inflammation, and increases insulin sensitivity—all great benefits that help support our goals. The World Health Organization (WHO) and Food and Agriculture Organization (FAO) both recommend a daily intake of at least 25 grams.[9] To gain the full benefits of fiber intake while doing keto, I recommend following their advice.

In practice, this means you eat up to 50 grams of total carbohydrates per day, sourced primarily from fibrous vegetables and fruits, such as leafy greens and berries. Fiber comes exclusively from plants. You don't have to track your fiber intake and align it perfectly on the dot to hit 25 grams (remember, we are humans dealing in averages, not machines). Simply shifting focus to unprocessed fibrous sources of carbs will help you achieve this goal.

Carbs on a Cyclical Keto Diet (CKD)

When it comes to carb cycling, our carbohydrate intake will exceed the appropriate amounts for a standard keto diet during certain meals or days. However, we aren't going to just tack extra carbs on top of our standard keto macros! Instead, we will swap out fat for carbs during high-carb meals and days. This allows protein needs to be met while shifting focus from one primary energy source to another to align with our TDEE, or determined deficit. In short, we'll eat the same number of calories as we would on an SKD but via carb-based meals instead of fat.

Gram for gram, carbs and fat do not provide equivalent energy. One gram of fat provides slightly more than double the calories that 1 gram of carbs contains; fat has 9 calories per gram, while carbs have only 4

Carb Goals for Cyclical Keto Diet (CKD)

Replace fat with carbs at a 1:2 ratio of fat to carb grams during high-carb meals.

calories per gram. When swapping carbs for fat, think of it as a 1:2 ratio of fat to carbs—for every gram of fat in your standard keto macros, you need to double the carb grams to get roughly the same amount of energy. We'll determine your standard keto fat macro in the next macronutrient section.

Let's say on a standard keto day, Amanda eats 80 grams of fat. Using the 1:2 fat to carb ratio, she can double the grams of carbs eaten on a high-carb day to 160 grams. This looks like double the calories, but it's not:

80 grams of fat = 720 calories (80 × 9 calories per gram = 720)

160 grams of carbs = 640 calories (160 × 4 calories per gram = 640)

Of course, Amanda can always do the math to get a more precise conversion, but the 1:2 ratio of fat to carbs is a quick way to determine a swap and allows a little wiggle room.

Performing the conversion calculation, we can see the caloric equivalent for 80 grams of fat is 180 grams of carbs:

80 grams of fat = 720 calories

720 calories ÷ 4 calories per gram of carbs = 180 grams of carbs

Of course, you don't have to meticulously track gram by gram. On a practical level, this swap from fat to carbs could simply involve choosing lean cuts of meat while minimizing cooking oil, butter, or other fatty condiments and incorporating high-carb ingredients with your protein sources. Selecting low-fat or no-fat options can help make the swap easier as well; instead of full-fat greek yogurt, grab the 0 percent fat variety. Simply being mindful to intentionally lower fat when you eat high-carb meals can help you naturally balance the calories without having to whip out a calculator, app, or kitchen scale every time you want to eat.

Once you begin eating keto, you will learn a lot about the nutrient content of your food and build confidence in your ability to select ingredients based on macronutrient content. This will make it much easier to intuitively cycle between low-carb and high-carb meals.

Carbs on a Targeted Keto Diet (TKD)

If you are incorporating a targeted keto diet strategy, your carbohydrate goals are going to look nearly identical to the SKD goals outlined previously except right before your workouts. On the days you perform high-intensity anaerobic exercise, you will add a small, targeted amount of quickly digested carbs 20 to 30 minutes before you ramp up your activity.

The amount of preworkout carbs to include ranges from 5 to 20 grams, though you can adjust as you see fit. If you are just transitioning or testing the waters between full-on standard keto and targeted keto to see how it affects your performance, I recommend starting at the lower end of the range, then gradually increasing as needed to find your sweet spot. If 5 grams of preworkout carbs doesn't make a difference but 20 grams makes you feel like a rock star, go with 20 grams of preworkout carbs! And if 20 grams isn't enough but 30 grams seems to make all the difference, don't feel constrained to the recommended ranges. This is your diet; you are the one putting in the work to get it on track and kick butt in the gym. Do what makes you feel best!

Because these carbs will be quickly burned up during your workout, feel free to use them as a supplement to your standard keto macros. In other words, you are not obligated to subtract your preworkout carbs from your allotted SKD carbs. Think of the preworkout carbs as a separate addition to your meals, a supplement to provide an extra boost!

Carbs on a Luteal Keto Diet (LKD)

The luteal keto diet (LKD) strategy merely aims to optimize the timing of your carbohydrate intake. During the follicular phase of your cycle, once you begin your menstrual bleed, you are primed for optimal carbohydrate metabolism. This is the best time to implement carb cycling, such as the cyclical keto diet (CKD) strategy, dispersing high-carb meals or days between the standard keto diet (SKD) strategy. Alternately, the follicular phase can be used as a time for continuous higher-carb eating—for example, a planned diet break.

Carb Goals for Targeted Keto Diet (TKD)

- Preworkout carbs: 5 to 20 grams before workout
- Total carb intake: Up to 50 grams daily + 5 to 20 grams preworkout carbs
- Dietary fiber intake: Target 25 grams daily
- Net carb intake: Up to 20 to 30 grams daily + 5 to 20 grams preworkout carbs

Carb Goals During Follicular Phase Using Luteal Keto Diet (LKD)

- High-carb meals/days: Replace fat with carbs at a 1:2 ratio in grams
- Total carb intake: Up to 50 grams daily
- Dietary fiber intake: Target 25 grams daily
- Net carb intake: Up to 20 to 30 grams daily

OR

- Plan a diet break

Carb Goals During Luteal Phase Using Luteal Keto Diet (LKD)

- Total carb intake: Up to 50 grams daily
- Dietary fiber intake: Target 25 grams daily
- Net carb intake: Up to 20 to 30 grams daily
- Preworkout carbs: 5 to 20 grams before workout as needed

During the luteal phase of the menstrual cycle, the time following ovulation, insulin sensitivity crashes as progesterone climbs, and appetite, cravings, and calories consumed all increase. This is not the best time for carb cycling or carb-based diets; this is the time to use a low-carb, standard keto diet to battle the adverse effects associated with this time of the month! Carbs during the luteal phase will remain low, using an SKD or TKD approach when appropriate.

Fat: Take It or Leave It

As for fat, we can take it or leave it. During low-carb, standard keto days, we'll definitely need to take it to meet our energy needs, but leaving it behind when eating high-carb meals will help us stay within our calorie goals. To put things into perspective, let's start with our standard keto macros.

Fat on a Standard Keto Diet: Take It

To figure out the amount of fat we should consume, we need to pull together our most basic body metrics: total daily energy expenditure (TDEE) and lean body mass.

Let's imagine your friend Jessica sees you reading this book. She admits she's confused about setting up her macros and asks for your help. You work with her to get all the appropriate measurements to determine her TDEE and lean body mass. Now what?

Jessica's TDEE: 2,200 calories
Jessica's lean body mass: 100 pounds (45.35 kg)

First, you will figure out how much protein Jessica needs to eat to support her lean mass. Being the insightful friend you are, you show her an acceptable range so she doesn't get hung up on any one specific number. Jessica is grateful to learn she needs between 60 and 100 grams of protein—she was under the impression she should limit her protein intake along with carbs. After watching her coworker, Julie, lose 5 pounds (2.25 kg) after drinking butter for a week, she thought that was the magic elixir behind keto. Yikes. You see where this is going and give Jessica the rundown on her lean mass before proceeding.

100 pounds lean mass × 0.6 g protein ÷ lb lean mass = 60 grams protein
100 pounds lean mass × 0.8 g protein ÷ lb lean mass = 80 grams protein
100 pounds lean mass × 1 g protein ÷ lb lean mass = 100 grams protein

You explain to Jessica that on a standard keto diet, carbohydrates are typically limited to under 50 grams, adequate protein intake supports lean mass (in her case 60 to 100 grams), and the rest of the body's energy needs are fueled by fat. After your chat, Jessica decides to aim for the middle of her adequate protein range to provide a convenient buffer in either direction. Now you're ready to calculate a well-rounded set of macros to get started. First, you will figure the maintenance levels for Jessica.

Fat calories = TDEE − protein calories − carb calories

TDEE = 2,200 calories

Protein calories = 80 grams protein × 4 calories per gram protein = 320 calories

Carb calories = 50 grams carbs × 4 calories per gram carb = 200 calories

Fat calories = 2,200 TDEE calories − 320 protein calories − 200 carb calories = 1,680 fat calories

Now, to calculate how many grams of fat this number of calories provides Jessica, you simply divide this number by 9:

Fat grams = 1,680 fat calories ÷ 9 calories per gram of fat = 186 grams of fat

Putting this data together provides Jessica with her maintenance-level macros for her current body composition and TDEE. If her goal is to maintain her weight while doing keto, she will need to eat roughly 50 grams of carbs, 80 grams of protein, and 186 grams of fat to fulfill her TDEE calorie requirements. When the caloric value of each macronutrient is compared against the total energy requirements for the day, we can see that carbs provide roughly 9 percent, protein 15 percent, and fat 76 percent. As discussed in chapter 1, maintenance keto macros are more aligned with what one would expect on a medically therapeutic keto diet.

But Jessica is not interested in maintaining her weight; she wants to get rid of excess body fat. You explain to Jessica that a calorie deficit is needed to tap into body fat stores for energy—her body won't burn them unless it has a reason to! Thanks to you, Jessica learns that because her carbohydrate intake is so low and her protein target is locked in to support lean mass, the only thing left to cut back on is dietary fat.

Jessica chooses a 25 percent calorie deficit, the upper end of the safe, moderate energy deficits. When Jessica asks whether she can go above 25 percent, you let her know that women with more weight to lose tend to tolerate higher levels of calorie restriction better. Jessica is free to play around with her calorie deficit to find what works and feels best, but you assure her that a 25 percent calorie restriction will deliver results and be sustainable long term. Now you calculate her new calorie goals and macros for fat loss.

TDEE = 2,200 calories

Calorie deficit = 2,200 calories × 25 percent = 550 calories

Daily calories at 25 percent deficit = 2,200 calories − 550 calories = 1,650 calories

Fat calories = 1,650 daily calories − 320 protein calories − 200 carb calories = 1,130 fat calories

Fat grams = 1,130 fat calories ÷ 9 calories per gram of fat = 125 grams of fat

To lose body fat with a 25 percent calorie deficit, Jessica's macros will be 50 grams of carbs, 80 grams of protein, and 125 grams of fat. Again, comparing Jessica's individual macronutrient goals to her body's daily energy needs, we can see the breakdown is as follows: 9 percent carbs, 15 percent protein, 51 percent dietary fat, and 25 percent body fat. The link between the calorie deficit and the portion of energy supplied by Jessica's body fat is apparent. Without the calorie deficit, the body would continue receiving all its energy needs from dietary sources and not burn any body fat.

Now, what if Jessica decided to join a gym and started regularly doing low- to moderate-intensity workouts? She would be better off with higher protein intake and bumping her protein ratio up to 1 gram per pound (454 g) of lean mass to help sustain her lean body composition. In turn, her fat macro would require adjustment to maintain her 25 percent calorie deficit.

Protein calories = 100 grams of protein × 4 calories per gram of protein = 400 calories

Fat calories = 1,650 daily calories − 400 protein calories − 200 carb calories = 1,050 fat calories

Fat grams = 1,050 fat calories ÷ 9 calories per gram of fat = 116 grams of fat

Jessica's macros would then be 50 grams of carbs, 100 grams of protein, and 116 grams of fat.

These calculated macros are not set in stone. They simply provide structure and guidance when choosing food to eat. Juggling three separate macronutrient goals, tallying them throughout the day, and worrying about hitting these numbers perfectly is not only stressful but also unnecessary. The stars don't need to align for you to be successful doing keto. You simply need to be in the ballpark, be mindful of what you eat, and adjust as you go based on your results and how you feel. Of course, there are fantastic tools to help count your macro intake for those who thrive on tracking (see page 174). But for all the women who feel great tracking, there are just as many women who struggle with this behavior. It can be overwhelming.

My suggestion is to target protein intake first and foremost, add slow-digesting carbs by way of fibrous veggies, and layer in the fat as needed, remembering that a little goes a long way. We'll discuss how to build easy keto meals in chapter 11.

Fat during High-Carb Meals or Days: Leave It
As carb intake increases, fat intake must decrease to accommodate the calorie shift. Think of a teeter-totter, with carbs on one end, fat on the other, and protein the fixed balance point in the middle. As carbs go up, fat goes down; as fat goes up, carbs go down. We are simply shifting the primary source of energy from one macro to another while ensuring we don't go overboard on calories. When carbs are high, we don't need much dietary fat. Focus on low-fat meals as you cycle in high-carb meals.

Remember, with cyclical keto we replace our standard keto fat grams with carb grams in a 1:2 fat to carb ratio, or, essentially, double our fat macro in grams to provide a relaxed frame of reference. Every gram of fat is swapped with 2 grams of carbs. Let's return to Jessica: She's been doing standard keto for several months, and after incorporating high-intensity exercise into her routine, she now feels like trying carb cycling one or two days a week.

Jessica's fat macro is 116 grams. On her high-carb days, she can eat the equivalent number of calories in carbs; doubling fat grams will give her a rough estimate. That means Jessica can eat 232 grams of carbs on her high-carb day, while keeping her fat low.

How low? Around the same number of calories that 50 grams of carbs provide on our standard, low-carb keto days. Just a simple swap. If we can double the grams of fat to arrive at an approximate high-carb equivalent, we can halve carb grams to arrive at a reasonably close fat equivalent. To do this, we simply take the standard 50 grams of carbs and cut it in half to get a fat macro for high-carb days. Though not an exact conversion, 25 grams of carbs would be an appropriate swap.

Alternately, do the extra calculations to arrive at more precise conversions between the two macronutrients, but it's certainly not required.

50 grams of carbohydrates × 4 calories per gram carbohydrate = 200 calories carbs

Fat grams = 200 calories ÷ 9 calories per gram of fat = 22.2 grams of fat

When eating high carb for the entire day, 20 to 25 grams of fat is a good target.

Although the gram conversion of 1:2 fat to carbs isn't perfect, I have found it close enough when dealing with the averages that come with diet and nutrition. As I mentioned before, the supplemental calculator tool for this book will make quick work of these items, and they perform the more precise conversions.

Again, using specific numbers and values isn't necessary. Building meals that are lean and low in fat during high-carb meals is sufficient to counter the high-carb intake.

So, we've learned that to help you get an estimate for energy needs and macronutrient goals during a keto diet for fat loss, use this book's supplemental calculator or manually follow the steps outlined here. Let's review.

Fat Goals for Cyclical Keto Diet (CKD)

Focus on minimizing fat intake while carbs are high.

Setting up macros for a standard keto diet is our first priority, as this serves as both the starting point for nutritional ketosis and "home base" for the other dieting strategies; when you aren't incorporating a carb-up, you will be eating this way. To do this, set your calorie requirements, based on TDEE and calorie deficit when appropriate. Next, determine your lean body mass to target a meaningful protein goal of 0.6 to 1 gram per pound (454 g) of lean mass. On a standard keto diet, carbohydrates are limited to a maximum of 50 grams, about half of which are fiber. Fat supplies the remainder of your energy needs, which can be formally calculated using your TDEE and calorie deficit, or guided intuitively based on hunger and satiety. Standard keto is what you will use to get into ketosis and become fat-adapted. If you choose to incorporate a carb-up strategy, standard keto will be what you return to immediately following to retain your fat-adapted metabolism.

When using the cyclical keto diet strategy, you will shift from higher fat intake to higher carb intake in a teeter-totter fashion. Fat intake will decrease as your carb intake increases. To determine macronutrient goals for cyclical keto, simply swap fat and carb macros by replacing the calories provided by fat on standard keto with carbs and vice versa. In grams, this is roughly equivalent to a 1:2 fat to carb ratio. Intuitively, you can achieve similar results by simply reducing fat intake during high-carb meals and days by choosing lower-fat ingredients.

The targeted keto diet strategy is nearly identical to the standard keto approach, only with the addition of quick-digesting preworkout carbs. Daily macronutrient goals do not change as a result of the preworkout; simply add on 5 to 20 grams of carbs to your standard keto macros and eat them about thirty minutes before your high-intensity workout.

The luteal keto diet is a mixture of the other three dieting strategies, focused on synchronizing carb-ups and continuous low-carb intake with the optimal times of your menstrual cycle. This strategy requires loosely tracking your hormonal cycle to initiate carb cycling strategies in the follicular phase and reverting back to continuous use of standard keto after ovulation during the luteal phase.

In the next chapter, you will learn the step-by-step approach to transitioning into nutritional ketosis, fat adaptation, and identifying problematic foods that interfere with your hormonal health and fat loss goals.

10

The Diet Phases

Throughout this book, I've presented so much information and so many suggestions and recommendations that by now you might be thinking, "Wow. That sounds like a lot! Can I really do this?" Yes, of course you can. But before we go any further, I want you to know you don't have to do it all at once.

In fact, small incremental steps are what I advocate for anyone trying to make lasting, long-term changes. It is unrealistic to expect someone to jump up and run a marathon after years of being glued to their couch, right? In the same way, it is unrealistic to expect anyone to go from not knowing how to cook or read a nutrition label to eating all organic, home-cooked meals perfectly aligned with their macronutrient goals. We need to take this one step at a time.

Now, I understand "one step at a time" may be a frustrating concept for those looking for quick fixes. But I don't really believe keto is an all-encompassing quick fix; if I did, this book would be a lot shorter: "Keep your carbs below 50 grams per day. The end." That's certainly an approach some take, and although it's not wrong, it's not necessarily optimal. In this chapter, I'm going to break down the components of the keto diet that we've discussed into more manageable, actionable steps. In addition to fat loss and improved hormonal balance, you'll build sustainable eating practices, learn a significant amount about the foods you eat, and understand what works best for your body by the time you reach the final steps.

The Dieting Phases

Phase 1: Getting Into Ketosis

Step 1: Tapering Carbs: 1 to 3 weeks

Step 2: Continuous Carb Restriction: 1 week

Step 3: Mastering Macros: 3 weeks

Phase 2: Fat-Adapted Living

Step 1: Testing the Waters: 1 meal

Step 2: Experimenting with Dieting Strategies: ongoing

Phase 3: Control-Alt-Delete

Step 1: Elimination: 3 weeks

Step 2: Reintroduction: ongoing

As written, the diet phases are intended to build slowly on each other, making small ongoing changes that lead to dramatic results. If you are already eating a keto diet and looking for ways to change your plan, feel free to jump to the section you find most applicable.

Phase 1: Getting into Ketosis

There are three major steps in this phase.

Step 1: Tapering Carbs

The purpose of tapering carbs is two-fold: gradually easing into carbohydrate restriction and developing a nutritional awareness of the food you eat. This step can last as long as you need it to; however, one to three weeks is generally sufficient.

When beginning keto, you can gently reduce carb intake over time or immediately drop to 50 grams of daily carbs—ripping off the bandage, so to speak. For women, especially those sensitive to thyroid issues, a more gradual approach to eliminating carbs is ideal. Our end goal will be limited to roughly 50 grams of carbs per day, and planning small daily decreases can get you to that number over a one to three week period. Perhaps you regularly eat 200 grams of carbs per day; dropping 10 grams of carbs each day will get you to ketogenic levels within a couple of weeks. At higher levels of carb intake, your daily decreases can also be higher, 15 to 30 grams. Alternately, set weekly reductions—a week one goal of 200 carb grams daily, followed by a second week at 150 grams, a third week at 100 grams, and finally our goal of 50 grams.

How you taper your carb intake will be based on how many carbs you currently eat and how long you plan to transition.

During this step, I want you to start a food journal to document your meals and beverages, taking note of pertinent nutrition information and ingredients. This process will help you develop mindful eating habits by becoming more aware of what and how much you eat, which is key to developing a healthy relationship with food. The practice of looking at nutrition information and ingredients will also help you become familiar with which foods are most appropriate for keto and which ones to avoid. You'll begin to notice macronutrient content when it may not have been something you paid much attention to.

The food journal can be an app if you'd like, but good old-fashioned pen and paper will work just fine. Putting pen to paper can help you retain the information, which can be beneficial as you learn appropriate food choices. The journal can also extend beyond the scope of logging food intake; it can be a place to document how certain foods make you feel, how you dealt with any frustrations or obstacles, or your thoughts about the process itself. Journaling can be a useful tool for stress management.

This step is extremely lax. There are no real restrictions and nothing is truly off limits. This is a time to acclimate and explore low-carb options without the pressure of following a prescribed diet, rules, or expectations; even the specifics of the carbohydrate taper are done on your terms, as you are ready.

Action Items

Start a food journal and write down all the food you eat, including nutrition information, each day. Gradually taper carbohydrate intake until you reach about 50 grams of carbohydrates daily; then you'll be ready to move on to the next step.

Step 2: Continuous Carb Restriction

Once you have reached a daily carbohydrate intake of around 50 grams, discontinue the taper. You made it! You're ready to make the transition into nutritional ketosis. Getting into ketosis requires a period of continuous carbohydrate restriction to fully deplete glycogen and encourage the body to produce ketones. Coming directly from a high-carbohydrate diet, this process generally takes several days; however, if you've been gradually fading out your carbohydrate intake, it may occur even faster. Physical activity also depletes glycogen, so exercise can help speed the process as well.

> The path to accelerated ketosis = very low carb intake + physical activity

Though nutritional ketosis will be achieved within several days of focused low-carb intake, give this step an entire week before moving on to the next stage. In fact, many keto dieters stop here, with limiting carbs as their one and only goal. Spend this week, or as much time as you need, adjusting to the lower carb intake. Get a feeling for how to manage it before adding another layer of complexity.

Continue documenting what you eat in your food journal. Are you eating real meals or are you munching on blocks of cheese, low-carb convenience bars, and pickles from the jar? Aside from limited carb intake, there are no restrictions for this step, but if you find yourself defaulting to precooked, low-carb convenience food, visit chapter 11 for some fresh ideas on building keto meals.

Step 3: Mastering Your Macros

This step focuses on aligning your nutrient goals with the foods you eat. Chapter 11 details several approaches to accomplishing this, including meal planning, tracking apps, and measuring methods. Continue to record meals in your food journal, making note of days that went well and those that didn't. Compare your meals to your macronutrient and calorie goals, looking for improvement opportunities and patterns in your eating behavior.

Ask yourself the following questions:

- What did I eat?
- When did I eat?
- Why did I eat?
- Am I staying within my carb limits?
- Am I eating enough protein?
- Am I over or under the calorie deficit I'm aiming for?
- What are my primary carb sources?
- What are my primary protein sources?
- What are my primary fat sources?
- Did this meal satisfy me?
- Is there anything that I should change or improve going forward?

Take time to reflect on your meals in this fashion as your body continues to develop adaptations for effective fat-burning. Continue this practice for several weeks to gain confidence

How to Tell whether You Are in Ketosis

There are a variety of tools on the market to indicate the presence of ketones, including urinary test strips, ketone breathalyzers, and ketone blood tests. Urinary ketone strips are a popular low-cost option that detect excess ketones spilled into the urine. In the initial stages of ketosis, these strips can serve as a visual indicator you are producing ketones, but they are not without issue. As the body begins relying on ketones for fuel, there are few to no excess ketones present in the urine, and as a result, the strips register negative. This sends the confusing message you are no longer in ketosis when you actually are; your body is just making positive adaptations to use ketones for fuel. The strips tend to be more useful in the beginning of carb restriction but lose their reliability over time. In my opinion, they are more of a nuisance than they are helpful.

Ketone breathalyzers measure ketone levels in the breath, and ketone blood meters test levels in the blood; they're similar to the devices diabetics use to test blood glucose levels. Of the three options, the blood meters offer the most accuracy. However, for fat loss purposes, monitoring ketone levels is unnecessary. Also, these devices can be expensive. Unless there is a medical necessity for measuring ketone levels or you are an inquisitive soul who must know for the sake of knowing, I don't recommend purchasing one.

My advice: Trust the process and save your money.

in your food choices. Over time, you will develop an intuitive connection between your food selections and dietary goals, which can help you become more mindful and intentional when you aren't actively tracking, planning, or measuring your food intake.

During these initial weeks of continuous carbohydrate restriction, your body will adjust and adapt your metabolism to rely on fatty acids and ketones for fuel rather than sugar. This can happen in as little as three weeks,[1] but for some it may take a bit longer. If you have been following the steps as outlined, your body will have had at least four weeks to switch from sugar-burner to fat-burner, and, by this time, fat adaptation either has been established or is well within reach.

What to Expect during Phase 1

In the beginning, expect to lose a fair amount of water weight as

How to Tell if You Are Fat-Adapted

Telltale signs of fat adaptation:

1. **The appetite suppressing effects of the keto diet have kicked in**. You can go for longer periods between meals without irritability or feeling the need to snack, without putting thought or effort into it.

2. **The brain fog and fatigue has lifted**. Even with adequate electrolyte supplementation, some people experience fatigue in the beginning stages of fat adaptation. You will feel more energy and mental clarity once fat-adapted.

3. **Low- to moderate-intensity workout performance has improved**. Physical activity can hit a slump after you start keto, but fat adaptation affords access to efficient fat-burning during exercise, so your slump should be over.

If any of these cues sounds familiar, feel free to move on to Phase 2. Alternately, continue in this phase indefinitely, sticking with the standard keto diet if you feel it suits you best. Regardless, I encourage you to consider Phase 3, where we aim to identify and eliminate problematic foods to reduce inflammation and support hormonal balance.

your glycogen stores are depleted and previously retained excess fluid is released. Over the several weeks of reduced carb intake, you may lose a fair bit of body fat as well! Even when you're not eating at an intentional calorie deficit, reduced hunger and increased satiety from eating foods low in carbs can naturally reduce your food intake and, in turn, your waistline.

One thing to be aware of during this time is the dreaded "keto flu." As you make the shift into ketosis, your body switches from hoarding sodium and water to getting rid of it in buckets, and potassium quickly follows suit. This leads to an electrolyte imbalance which, if not corrected, can leave you feeling downright awful. Headaches that won't quit, dizziness, shakiness, fatigue, irritability, cramping, constipation, and wow my brain hurts just thinking about it. If you've dropped your carbs for a couple of days and suddenly feel like crawling into bed for all eternity, don't panic. The electrolyte imbalance, or "keto flu," can easily be corrected, or prevented altogether (see page 177).

Phase 2: Fat-Adapted Living

In phase 2, we'll test the waters and experiment with dieting strategies.

Step 1: Testing the Waters

By now, you've been restricting carbohydrates for some time. Although many women are eager to start incorporating more carbs into their diet with light carb cycling, preworkout carbs, or full-on high-carb days, others struggle to warm up to the idea after seeing such great results doing a standard keto diet. It can require a bit of a mind-set shift.

This step is intended to break the ice between your extended period of carb restriction and implementation of the dieting strategies discussed in chapter 8 for those who choose to incorporate them. It's just one high-carb meal, arguably the easiest step of all. Testing the waters with a single high-carb meal can help you assess whether you are ready to experiment with strategic carb intake.

If you feel prepared, move on to the next step.

However, if you are concerned that all your progress will unravel with temporary high-carb intake or fear that this one high-carb meal will extend into a monthlong carb bender, don't feel obligated to do something you aren't comfortable with or ready for. Your concerns are legitimate and extremely common. Sticking with a standard keto diet may be your best bet for now.

Step 2: Experimenting with Dieting Strategies

Once you've reached this step, it's time to decide which alternative dieting strategy to pursue. This will largely be determined based on your goals, physical activity, and menstrual cycle. This step is more of an ongoing process as you experiment and tailor the diet to meet your needs. Refer back to chapter 8 to guide your decision and implementation.

What to Expect During Phase 2

If you are using CKD for hormonal balance and fat loss, expect thyroid levels to improve, stress hormones to drop, and your metabolic rate to increase to keep your fat loss goals on the right track. If you've chosen to use CKD or TKD for athletic purposes, expect your performance to improve. If you've decided to home in on your menstrual cycle to optimize your diet with the LKD, expect to reap all the benefits of the CKD in the first phase of the cycle, while leveraging standard keto in the second phase to fight off wild cravings and raging appetite to continue losing fat.

Phase 3: Control-Alt-Delete

In phase 3, we'll encounter elimination and reintroduction.

Step 1: Elimination

An important piece of the hormonal balance and weight loss puzzle involves reducing inflammation and repairing gut health. Although a standard keto diet does a bang-up job of this, some low-carb foods that support nutritional ketosis can actually work *against* these efforts. Unfortunately, many women have unknown underlying food allergies, sensitivities, and intolerances that can trigger inflammation, interfering with their mission to balance hormones and lose weight. Phase 3, or what I like to call the "Control-Alt-Delete" phase, aims to reset your diet to a clean slate so you can easily identify foods that trigger a negative response.

This is a beneficial step for everyone to include in their diet plan, but women with continued inflammation, chronic headaches, digestive issues such as constipation or bloating, and skin issues such as acne and eczema will find especially great benefit. It is also particularly helpful for women who have experienced a weight loss stall for an extended time.

A big red flag of underlying food sensitivity or intolerance is digestive issues following a high-carb meal, if you have started incorporating them into your diet strategy. It's likely not the carbs but one of the ingredients in something you ate.

This is an opportunity to give your body a rest from a constant flux of potentially inflammatory ingredients and observe how your body responds once they are reintroduced. This will help you further home in on the foods that optimize your health, while avoiding foods that cause negative symptoms in your body.

To begin the elimination step, omit the following ingredients from your diet for a minimum of three weeks:

- Alcohol
- Artificial sweeteners
- Dairy
- Soy
- Wheat/gluten

This is not an exhaustive list of all potential allergens, but it includes the most common triggers known to cause inflammation, result in hormonal imbalance, and impair weight loss efforts. If you suspect there are other ingredients causing issues, omit them as well. You know your body better than anyone. Perhaps someone has convinced you that something you like to eat is "not keto," citing inflammatory reasons; if you want to investigate whether it actually applies to you, add it to the list. Naturally, if you are already aware of ongoing allergens, food sensitivities, and intolerances, do not include those foods in your diet at any point.

I have included this process in the final implementation phase of the diet, guiding your efforts to improve continuously on your diet. Of course, you can avoid these potential problem ingredients from the beginning, if you choose, or perform an elimination phase prior to starting keto.

Step 2: Reintroduction

The reintroduction step is exactly what it sounds like: You reintroduce the previously eliminated foods. Not all at once, though. Try one thing at a time, observe the effects (if any), and proceed. There is no time limit on this step, as reintroducing food should be done at your convenience, when you have the best opportunity to pay attention to the symptoms your body is sending. And, of course, during a time you are prepared to deal with any potentially negative symptoms. Don't load up on dairy right before a hot date, if you get my drift.

Your food journal will be your best friend during this process. If you haven't diligently been documenting what you're eating since phase 1, now is the time to start. Record your meals, including ingredients, and document any negative effects in the period that follows. Recording this reintroduction step can also provide insight into how your current diet compares to your initial weeks on keto. Chances are you've improved your diet by leaps and bounds.

Here's what it will look like in practice:

> Day 1: Reintroduce one ingredient. Observe and document any symptoms that follow immediately and throughout the rest of the day.

> Days 2 to 3: Abstain from the ingredient and continue to observe and record any symptoms.

Some symptoms may be more obvious than others, which is why I suggest picking a time when you can get in tune with your body. Symptoms may include diarrhea, acne breakouts, bloating, flatulence, rashes, sleep issues, migraines, tension headaches, ringing in the ears, stomach cramps, constipation, indigestion, muscle aches, joint pain, and mood swings—to list a few. Again, you know your body best. If anything is out of the ordinary, take note.

Maybe you experienced one of these symptoms but aren't quite sure the ingredient was the culprit. Take it back out of your diet and retest to confirm.

If you reintroduce an ingredient and don't experience anything but a delicious meal, then keep it in your diet, feeling confident you tolerate it well.

What to Expect During Phase 3

As you eliminate certain ingredients in the first step of phase 3, you may notice decreased bloating, improved digestion, reduced inflammation, clearer skin, migraine or headache relief, and further weight loss if any of the eliminated foods previously caused these symptoms in your body. If you've been living with food your body doesn't agree with, it can feel like a weight has been lifted! While you can expect some temporary discomfort in the reintroduction phase if you run into problematic ingredients, you will now have peace of mind that you are eating the best foods for *your* body.

Before moving on, let's review what we just learned. Phase 1 is intended to ease you into ketosis and get your body to burn fat effectively as its preferential source of energy. Steps 1, 2, and 3 of the initial phase embody the basics of a standard keto diet for women. Continue here, move to the next phase, or skip ahead to phase 3, depending on your goals.

Phase 2 is all about tailoring the standard keto diet to meet your needs and optimizing hormonal balance.

And, finally, phase 3 focuses on personalizing the diet to your unique nutritional needs by systematically identifying problem foods that cause inflammation, hormonal imbalance, and stalled weight loss.

In the next chapter, we will begin connecting the dots between your macronutrient goals, dieting strategies, and all the delicious foods you can enjoy on the keto diet.

11

Keto Food Literacy

"What should I eat?" Ah, the question that plagues every new dieter. When you are just getting started, trying to identify which foods are most compatible with keto and how much to eat can feel like a daunting task. Don't get discouraged. This chapter is all about the tasty foods you can enjoy on a keto diet: optimal foods to eat, what foods to avoid, how to determine the nutritional content of your food, and different approaches to align your meals with your nutrient goals.

Think back to chapter 3, where we discussed conflicting food values. Remember, carbo-hydrate restriction alone determines the metabolic state of nutritional ketosis, not necessarily a list of foods or particular ingredients. This is a friendly reminder that anything low enough in carbohydrates can support nutritional ketosis. As such, there are not really keto vs. nonketo foods. Just about anything can fit with a keto diet if you take small enough nibbles, slice it thin enough, or bury it deep within an ingredients list.

That said, not every food is an excellent choice for optimizing nutrient density and hormonal balance, even if it technically supports ketosis. Do hot dogs and pasture-raised pork both support keto? Yes. Are they nutritionally equivalent? Of course not.

With that in mind, I will provide food options and recommendations targeted on boosting nutrition to align with the overarching goals of this book. These are not "rules" or conclusive lists; they are simply examples and suggestions to get you started and guide your food choices.

Most foods have a mixed macronutrient composition. This means there is a combination of three different macronutrient groups contributing to the overall energy provided and, in turn, your macros. Take an avocado: The fruit has a high fat content but also provides a source of carbohydrates (namely fiber) and protein. Nuts are a high-fat food with both protein and carbs. Fatty cuts of meat contain both protein and fat, while even lean meats may contain small amounts of fat. When I talk about protein, fat, and carb sources, please note the foods generally provide a combination of the three.

Protein Sources

You may think of meat when you hear protein, but there are actually meat, seafood, and vegetarian sources.

Meat and Seafood

Meat and fish are both very low in carbohydrates and are high-quality protein sources, meaning they provide all the essential amino acids from these foods. Although the macronutrient content of meat and fish is primarily protein, some cuts of meat and certain kinds of fish also contain a good amount of fat. Similarly, while protein based, some shellfish also supply carbohydrates. The skin of meat and fish is high in fat. If you are intentionally keeping fat intake lower to align with a calorie deficit or dieting strategy, taking the skin off or choosing lean proteins can help you do that. Organ meats can be an excellent source of nutrients suitable for ketogenic diets as well.

Not all meat is raised equally; its quality and nutritional content is affected by the environment, treatment, and food the animals receive. Many animals are raised with hormones and antibiotics, which increases our own exposure and can affect our hormonal balance. When farm animals are fed foods they aren't intended to eat and their physical activity is limited, the nutrient content of their meat suffers. Think of what has happened to the human population over the years as we began eating foods not intended for our biology and reduced our physical activity; we became riddled with disease. Do you want to eat food like that or food from animals that have been provided optimal diet and exercise?

Pasture-raised animals provide many nutritional benefits not afforded by feedlot-raised animals. The meat of grass-fed animals is higher in anti-inflammatory omega-3 fatty acids than that of grain-fed animals. The fat in animals raised on grain is mainly omega-6 fatty acids. Additionally, the meat and eggs of free-range poultry have higher omega-3 content than the alternative.

Examples of Protein from Meat and Seafood

Beef	Goat	Quail
Bison	Goose	Rabbit
Chicken	Lamb	Salmon
Clam	Lobster	Scallop
Crab	Mussel	Shrimp
Deer	Oyster	Trout
Duck	Pheasant	Tuna
Eggs	Pork	Turkey

Why does this matter? The human body has evolved to have a 1:1 ratio of omega-3 to omega-6 fats.[1] In our body, these two fats have opposing functions and compete for the same enzymes to complete their biochemical reactions.[2] When we eat excessive amounts of omega-6, we create a nutrient imbalance that alters metabolic pathways. Omega-3's anti-inflammatory path is shut down, and the production of inflammatory arachidonic acid and eicosanoids is triggered.[3] By eating foods high in omega-6, we can easily take in excess and activate inflammation in our bodies. When meat is our primary protein source, as often is the case on a keto diet, we can be susceptible to this if we aren't diligent about choosing higher-quality animal products.

Omega-3 fatty acids have also been shown to be of particular benefit to women's health, balancing hormones and preventing health complications. Studies have shown omega-3 consumption is beneficial for improving or preventing the following:

- Breast cancer[4]
- Depression[5]
- Hot flashes during menopause transition[6]
- Menstrual pain[7]
- Osteoporosis[8]
- Irregular menstrual cycles[9]
- Excess testosterone levels in women[10]

The take-home point: Focus on including higher omega-3 content by selecting properly raised animal products when you can; choose organic and pasture-raised meats and wild-caught seafood.

Vegetarian Protein Sources

It can be challenging to find high-quality, complete protein sources suitable for a vegetarian keto diet, but there are options. Eggs are a popular nonmeat source of protein that offers a complete amino acid profile. Chicken and duck eggs are both fantastic vegetarian choices. If your macronutrient goals require you to reduce fat intake, egg whites are a nearly fat-free choice of protein.

Tofu is also an option for those who include soy in their diet. It can be used as a meat substitute in a variety of dishes and is also a complete source of amino acids. If you do incorporate tofu into your keto diet to target protein, choose the firmer varieties, as they generally have a higher protein content.

If you tolerate dairy, protein can also be found in cheeses and yogurts. Plain, strained greek yogurt can provide a substantial amount of protein, and the fat-free varieties can help you balance your macros as needed. Cheese can also serve to fill your protein needs; however, many are primarily fat based, and the calories can add up quickly. Cottage cheese, both regular and dry curd, is another source that offers both high- and low-fat options.

Examples of Vegetarian Protein Sources

Cheese	Nuts
Eggs, whole	Seeds
Egg whites	Tofu
Greek yogurt, plain	Vegetables

Additionally, many plant sources of protein can be enjoyed on a keto diet. Nuts, seeds, and some vegetables contain protein that can contribute to your daily macronutrient goal. When choosing plant-based sources of protein, remember most are not complete proteins and will be missing key amino acids. Include a variety of sources such as almonds, chia seeds, cottage cheese, broccoli, and mushrooms to ensure a complete amino acid profile in your diet. While legumes are a source of protein, they are often high in carbohydrates and are not suitable for standard keto diets. Soybeans, green beans, and peanuts are exceptions and can be eaten on the diet.

Again, when choosing animal products, such as dairy or eggs, selecting the organic and pasture-raised options can help promote hormonal balance and prevent inflammation.

Fat Sources

Now let's look at potential sources for the fat your diet needs.

Fats and Oils

As your macronutrient goals determine the upper limit for your fat consumption, it is essential to pay attention to the quantities you use. Remember, fat is the most calorically dense of the macronutrients; unlike most other foods, oils and fats are composed of just one single macronutrient, which contains 9 calories per gram. Even small amounts of these ingredients carry loads of energy. Measure the fats and oils you use to cook and include with your meals, rather than drizzling them all over with reckless abandon.

Going overboard on fats and oils can lead to increased calorie consumption. If you regularly exceed your calorie needs, you will not lose fat despite being in nutritional ketosis. Ketosis does not equal fat loss—a negative energy balance does. And perhaps even more importantly, ketosis is not bulletproof protection against weight gain if you regularly overdo it on calories.

The point is fat is not a "free food" simply because you are doing keto. You need fat to fuel your energy requirements; going above and beyond that will not help your cause.

When selecting the best fats and oils, there are three primary things to consider: how they are made, their chemical makeup, and their smoke point.

Vegetable Oils High in Omega-6

Canola oil	Rice-bran oil
Corn oil	Sesame oil
Cottonseed oil	Soybean oil
Peanut oil	Sunflower oil

Choosing oils that are less processed will help maintain their nutrition and natural antioxidants; refining processes strip them of these benefits. When you can, select cold-pressed oils, also known as "virgin" oils, for maximum nutritional value. Additionally, fats that hail from hormone-free, pasture-raised animals will yield a higher quality product nutritionally.

To prevent inflammation, it's important to reduce omega-6 sources in favor of omega-3 fats to balance our body's ideal ratio. Certain oils are high in omega-6, which can tilt the scales in favor of metabolic pathways that produce inflammatory molecules that wreak havoc in the body. This goes double when eaten in higher quantities afforded by keto diet macros. Does that mean you can't have them at all? No, but you should look elsewhere for your primary fat sources and cooking oils.

Also relevant to the chemical makeup of fats and oils is whether they are saturated. This becomes more important when used for cooking. Saturated fats are generally those that are solid at room temperatures while unsaturated fats tend to remain liquid. Saturated fats are more stable when cooking due to their chemical structure, while unsaturated fats are susceptible to oxidation when exposed to high heat and can form free radicals during the cooking process.[11] A lower temperature is preferable when cooking with unsaturated cooking oils.

Free radicals are unstable, highly reactive atoms due to unpaired electrons in their outer shell. In a quest to pair the electrons for stability, they seek out other atoms and molecules to bind to in the body, which can trigger a domino-like effect of electron stealing, causing damage to cells, proteins, and DNA. This is known as "oxidative stress," which can lead to chronic inflammation and contribute to a host of other disorders. Free radicals are one reason eating foods rich in antioxidants is so important. Antioxidants squelch free radicals, preventing them from stealing electrons from critical sources and causing damage.

The smoke point of fats and oils is also important when cooking. The smoke point is the temperature at which your oil goes from a beautiful sizzling sheen in the pan to setting off your smoke detector. Those clouds of smoke aren't just annoying; they are an indication that your oil is degrading and releasing free radicals. If you are going to cook with fats, consider the temperature you'll be working with.

Special Consideration: MCT Oils

Medium-chain triacylglycerols, also known as MCTs, are a favorite fat source among keto dieters. Due to their chemical structure, MCTs are more quickly digested and absorbed directly into the bloodstream. This is in contrast to the long, drawn-out digestion of long

FATS SAFE FOR HIGH-HEAT COOKING[12]		
Ingredient	Saturated Fat Content	Smoke Point
Butter	High	Medium to High
Coconut oil	High	Medium to High
Beef fat	High	High
Ghee	High	High
Palm oil	High	High
Pork fat	Medium	High
Duck fat	Medium	High
FATS SAFE FOR LOW-HEAT COOKING		
Avocado oil	Low	High
Macadamia nut oil	Low	High
Olive oil	Low	High

chain triacylglycerols. That makes MCTs a great source of rapidly available energy for those who need it and a way to amplify ketone levels. Ketogenic athletes of all kinds may find MCTs a useful tool for fueling workouts without relying on carbohydrates. Natural sources of MCTs primarily include coconut and palm oil. Most commercially available MCT products have extracted the MCT fatty acids from one of these two sources and condensed them into supplement form.

Nuts and Seeds

Nuts and seeds are plant-based sources of fat that are full of nutrients, including fiber, magnesium, and vitamin E. Nuts and seeds are the types of foods that contain a blend of macronutrients; while they are listed under fat sources, they are also a source of protein and carbohydrates.

Examples of Nuts and Seeds

Almonds	Hazelnuts	Sesame seeds
Almond butter	Hemp seeds	Sunflower seeds
Almond flour	Macadamias	
Almond meal	Macadamia butter	Sunflower seed butter
Brazil nuts	Pecans	Sunflower seed flour
Cashews	Pine nuts	Tahini
Cashew butter	Pistachios	Walnuts
Coconut	Pumpkin seeds	
Coconut flour		

A Note about Trans Fats

Cis and *trans* are terms used to describe how unsaturated fatty acids are arranged. The cis form is the most naturally occurring form, while only small amounts of trans fats exist in nature. Most trans fatty acids are artificially produced by food manufacturers. Trans fats have a solid texture, similar to saturated fats, but their shelf life extends well beyond any naturally occurring fats. Commercially, this allows processed foods to sit on the shelf without spoiling. Nutritionally? Absolutely awful.

In 2015, the U.S. Food and Drug Administration placed an official ban on adding artificial trans fats to manufactured food after making a final determination that artificial trans fats were no longer to be generally recognized as safe in human food.[13] In 2018, the World Health Organization announced a plan to eradicate industrially produced trans-fatty acids from the global food supply.[14] A massive win throughout the world! However, there is an allowed grace period for compliance from manufacturers; check food labels if you purchase processed foods susceptible to the addition of trans fat.

It is wise to portion your nuts and seeds to avoid carbs and calories creeping up. Whole nuts and seeds make easy, delicious foods, but without thoughtful portioning, they can become an exercise in mindless eating, racking up calories and carbs without you being fully in tune with how much you are eating. Similarly, nut butters have very high energy and nutrient density. A little goes a long way! Measuring appropriate serving sizes rather than spooning almond butter straight from the container will help you achieve your fat loss goals.

There are quite a few flours made from nuts and seeds that can be used in place of high-carb wheat flour. Gravies, sauces, and low-carb baked goods, such as bread, cookies, and pizza dough, are just a few of the creative way to use these low-carb flours. These types of recipes are great for special occasions on a standard keto diet, but they are not diet staples. Keep it simple, stick with whole foods, and the results will pay off!

Dairy

If tolerated, certain types of dairy can also be enjoyed on the keto diet. If you suspect a dairy intolerance or are not sure, consider trying an elimination period to find out (see page 151). Some dairy can be relatively high in carbohydrates due to the lactose, or milk sugar, content. The higher the fat content of the dairy food, the fewer carbohydrates there are. For example, a glass of nonfat milk has higher carbs than whole milk, while heavy cream has far less than both.

Additionally, many low-fat or fat-free dairy items contain added sugars and starches to improve flavor and consistency, which increase overall carb count. It's best to watch the ingredient labels if you choose to include dairy in your diet.

At risk of sounding like a broken record, I urge you to choose organic and pasture-raised dairy options when available. The hormones used to raise nonorganic dairy cows transfer into the milk, triggering effects that alter our own biological processes and hormone balance.[15]

Carb Sources

Keto-friendly sources of carbohydrates include vegetables and legumes, fruits, and spices.

Vegetables and Legumes

One thing that nutrition experts agree on is that vegetables are an essential part of a healthy, nutrient-dense diet. However, not all plant-based foods are inherently low in carbohydrates, which can add to the initial confusion about what to eat on a standard keto diet. You absolutely can eat vegetables on a keto diet, and I encourage you to do so for the vitamins, minerals, and beneficial bioactive compounds that maximize your overall nutrition.

Determining which vegetables are conducive to nutritional ketosis in higher quantities largely depends on the fiber and starch content. In general, stay away from high-starch vegetables and lean toward those with higher fiber content. In other words, we are looking for low-sugar plants when we choose our vegetables.

Examples of Keto-Friendly Dairy Products

Blue cheese	Cream cheese	Mozzarella cheese
Brie	Feta cheese	
Butter	Ghee	Parmesan cheese
Cheddar cheese	Goat cheese	
Colby jack cheese	Gouda cheese	Provolone cheese
	Greek yogurt, plain	Ricotta
Cottage cheese		Sour cream
	Heavy whipping cream	Swiss cheese

Examples of Keto-Compatible Vegetables

Alfalfa sprouts	Celery	Nori
Artichoke	Chard	Okra
Arugula	Chicory greens	Radish
Asparagus	Collard greens	Romaine lettuce
Beet greens	Endive	
Bok choy	Escarole	Rutabaga
Broccoli	Green beans	Seaweed
Broccoli rabe	Iceberg lettuce	Spinach
Brussels sprouts	Jicama	Turnip
Bibb lettuce	Kohlrabi	Water spinach
Butter lettuce	Mung beans	
Cabbage	Mushrooms	
Cauliflower	Mustard greens	

Leafy greens are excellent low-starch, high-fiber vegetables. Keeping the color green in mind can be a helpful guideline when in doubt. Much like a traffic light, green means go! Though of course, that is more of a generalization than a rule. The truth is many other vegetables fit within the framework of a standard keto diet; including a wide variety will help maximize the nutrient density of your diet for optimal health. As you proceed, you'll develop increased confidence making selections.

Starch-rich vegetables tend to grow underground as roots and tubers or aboveground in pods—think legumes. Roots and tuber vegetables that have relatively high carb content include yuca, yams, potatoes, and carrots. Legumes that are high in carbs include beans, lentils, and peas. But even these guidelines are not hard and fast rules. Radishes, turnips, and jicama are root vegetables with low carbohydrate content. Green beans and peanuts are legumes that can easily coexist with a standard keto diet. Starchy vegetables can still be enjoyed on a standard keto diet in moderation with mindful portion sizes. And as you become fat-adapted, you can include them more frequently and in more substantial amounts.

Beware of Juice and Dehydrated Fruits

When fruits are juiced, most of the fiber is stripped from the final product. As a result, you are left with a highly concentrated sugary beverage that will dramatically affect your blood sugar and insulin response and affect nutritional ketosis if consumed in large enough amounts. The exceptions are lemon and lime juice, which can be used in moderation due to their relatively low sugar content compared to other fruit juices.

When moisture is removed from fruits during the dehydration process, the fruit becomes more nutrient dense than its fresh counterpart. Consequently, this means higher carb and sugar count by weight. For example, in 100 grams (3½ ounces) of raw apricot, there are roughly 11 grams of carbohydrates. But in 100 grams of dehydrated apricot, the carb count skyrockets to 82 grams.[16] The difference is significant, and you will find similar trends with other dried or dehydrated fruits, including prunes, raisins, and fruit leather.

Knowing that vegetables have carbs, some people avoid them altogether, aiming for zero carb intake or something akin to a "carnivore" diet. Although it may be an effective strategy for some, avoiding plants altogether can put you at risk of nutrient deficiencies if you are not obtaining the lost nutrients from other sources. It's not something I personally recommend, especially over long periods.

Fruits

Fruits are often avoided on standard keto diets because many are high carb by nature. But that doesn't mean you can't have fruit. Just as we did with vegetables, we can seek out low-sugar plants to point us in the right direction.

By choosing fruits low in sweetness, high in fiber, and often mistaken for vegetables, you can actually incorporate a healthy diversity on a standard keto diet.

Fruits that are either tart or savory tend to have lower amounts of natural sugar, which translates to a relatively low overall carbohydrate count. Lemon is an excellent example—it's less sweet but can be incorporated into many dishes. Olives are an example of a savory fruit that fits perfectly within the structure of a standard keto diet.

As previously discussed, fiber is largely unabsorbed and, therefore, does not affect nutritional ketosis. High-fiber fruits, such as berries and avocado, may appear high in total carbohydrates, but the carbs from fiber are less impactful on your metabolic state and contribute very little to calorie intake. These types of fruits can also be enjoyed on a standard keto diet.

And, of course, many fruits that are often considered vegetables can be enjoyed on a standard keto diet. These are otherwise known as low-carb vegetables that are technically fruits. Tomatoes, tomatillos, avocados, zucchini—pretty much any seed-bearing vegetable you can think of—those "veggies" are fruits, botanically speaking. This point is less about debating what constitutes a fruit or vegetable and more about breaking free from the "no fruit on keto" mind-set. Most keto dieters eat plenty of fruit, even if they aren't aware it's technically a fruit.

Examples of Keto-Compatible Fruits

Avocado	Cucumber	Raspberry
Banana pepper	Eggplant	Rhubarb
Bell pepper	Gooseberry	Spaghetti squash
Blackberry	Grapefruit	
Black olive	Green olive	Strawberry
Boysenberry	Jalapeño pepper	Summer squash
Carambola a.k.a. starfruit		Tomatillo
	Lemon	
Casaba melon	Lime	Tomato
Chayote	Oheloberry	Zucchini
Coconut	Prickly pear	

Spices

Spices are a great way to improve the flavor of your food and provide many beneficial compounds that enhance health and nutrition. Most spices are primarily carbohydrate based, but because they are used in such small quantities—a teaspoon in an entire recipe or an extra dash for good measure—in the grand scheme of things, spices are often negligible.

However, carbohydrates do have the potential to add up if you are extremely heavy handed in your use. In practice, you can count the macros from spices or be laxer with your seasonings. Let the size of the meal and overall portions guide your decision. There is little value in being meticulous about pinches and sprinkles, but consider the contribution to your macros in more copious amounts.

That said, some spices have extra ingredients. Many include sugar, starches, or other fillers in addition to the advertised spice. Spice mixes and seasoning packets are notorious for this, and the carbohydrates can be surprisingly high—for example, 18 grams in a small package of taco seasoning![17] When possible, avoid commercial spice mixes and make your own. You can get a great idea of the main spices included in your favorite blends by peeking at the ingredients list on the nutrition label.

A Note about High-Carb Foods

As discussed in chapter 2, whether eating low carb or high carb, consume refined carbohydrates or added sugars sparingly. They offer poor nutritional value and have been identified as the primary contributors to the modern obesity and diabetes epidemic. Luckily, the framework of a standard keto diet doesn't offer room for these types of foods. By shopping for the minimally processed whole food ingredients listed in the previous sections, you will likely avoid refined carbohydrates and sugars altogether.

On a standard keto diet, avoiding sugars, starches, and grains will help keep carbohydrates low. However, if you transition into a cyclical keto diet or targeted keto diet, your dietary options widen to include the very things you diligently abstained from. What should you choose? Are all sugars, starches, and grains created equal?

Cyclical Keto Diet Carbs

On days you include higher levels of carbohydrates in your diet, I encourage you to continue sourcing the majority of carbs from vegetable and fruit sources. Enjoy nutrient-dense sweet potatoes, yams, carrots, winter squash, and beets. Legumes, such as lentils, chickpeas, or black beans, are fair game. Your fruit options expand to include the sweeter varieties: bananas, plantains, persimmons, and figs. Keep your diet focused on whole, nutrient-dense foods with minimal processing when you cycle in high-carb meals or days.

These meals can include unrefined grains as well—whole grains, such as whole-wheat products, multigrain bread, and oats—if you tolerate them and they align with your personal food values. If you have a gluten allergy or intolerance, you can still enjoy quinoa, teff, millet, wild rice, brown rice, and buckwheat (despite its somewhat misleading name).

I encourage you to continue making healthful dietary choices during your high-carb meals. Remember, they are a strategy to help you reach your goals, not an excuse to eat junk food.

Targeted Keto Diet Carbs

For TKD preworkout carbs, you want to use quickly digested sources of carbohydrates that will be made available to the muscles. For best results, minimize fructose intake. Fructose is, essentially, trapped in the liver after absorption. Not only does this interfere with ketosis for more extended periods, but it also prevents the muscles from getting the energy needed during the high-intensity workout. It's simply not a useful fuel for TKD purposes.

I recommend avoiding high-fructose corn syrup altogether; not only is it concentrated fructose, but it also contributes to insulin resistance and increases lipogenesis, the process of converting carbohydrates directly into fat.[18] Agave syrup is another very high-fructose food to avoid for this purpose.

Most fruits have a mix of glucose and fructose sugars in a roughly 50/50 ratio, as does honey. Coconut sugar and maple syrup are primarily sucrose sugars, disaccharides composed of equal parts glucose and fructose. Most natural sugar sources contain at least some fructose. Though they do contain fructose, any of these options is a better alternative to agave or high-fructose corn syrup.

Whole grains are generally fructose free, but they tend to digest more slowly. Quickly digested refined grains, on the other hand, often contain high-fructose corn syrup. Rice is both fructose free and a quickly absorbed grain, making it suitable for TKD purposes. High glycemic index starchy vegetables with lower fiber content tend to be more rapidly digested as well—they include yams, peas, parsnips, sweet potato, and white potato.

As you can see, there are whole food options for this purpose, though some may choose more refined alternatives.

Fruits with More Glucose than Fructose[19]

Apricot	Date	Peach
Banana	Fig, dried	Plum
Cherry	Nectarine	Prune

Keto-Friendly Sweeteners

Erythritol	Monk fruit	Stevia

Low-Carb Beverages

Almond milk	Cashew milk	Herbal tea
Broth and stock	Coconut milk	Macadamia milk
Carbonated water*	Coffee	
	Hemp milk	

*Tonic water is an exception due to the high sugar content

Ultimately, you will roughly be eating 5 to 20 grams of carbs for this purpose, which, in most cases, is less than a whole serving of anything listed. Regardless of what you choose, preworkout carbs will help your high-intensity exercise performance during a TKD. Lyle McDonald, exercise physiologist and author of *The Ketogenic Diet*, explains that "a wide variety of foods have been used prior to workouts: glucose polymers, SweeTarts, bagels, and food bars; all result in improved performance" on a targeted ketogenic diet.[20]

Miscellaneous

My focus has been on whole foods, so as to avoid over-complicating things. However, there are other things that can be enjoyed on a keto diet, such as certain sweeteners and various beverages. When in doubt, read the label!

Keto-Friendly Sweeteners

The sweeteners listed in the sidebar above are all-natural, low-carb, and low glycemic index sugar replacements. When counting "net" carbs, dieters often subtract these from their daily carbohydrate count in addition to fiber due to their minimal impact on blood sugar and lack of calorie content. However, sweeteners may not be tolerated by everyone, as they are known to cause digestive upset and bloating in some.

Low-Carb Beverages

The beverages listed to the left are all low in carbohydrates and suitable for a standard keto diet. Many can also be used as liquids for cooking. Please note each option is unsweetened. Check the labels to ensure the brands you select are truly low in carbohydrates.

Food Labels and Beyond

Nutrition-label literacy is a valuable skill, especially when on a fat loss mission. The information on nutrition labels can help guide your choices at the grocery store and help keep tabs on what you eat throughout the day. Although the calorie and macronutrient data will be your key focus to remain within the general keto framework, there's a plethora of information packed into those little tables. As I warned previously, nutrition data is often based on averages, estimates, and what is found to be reasonably accurate. Nutrition labeling laws differ from country to country, but in the United States, all values are rounded to the nearest whole number. By U.S. food labeling laws, any macronutrient less than 0.5 grams per serving can be rounded down to zero. This is not a huge deal but can be confusing when you start looking at labels listing zero only to find out later they can contribute to your overall carb count.

Here's a step-by-step primer on reading a nutrition label:

1. **Check the serving size.** This gives you a clear understanding of what the rest of the data mean. Can you eat the whole package, or is it actually divvied into six minuscule portions? Then you can decide whether that's a realistic amount to eat and whether the carb count fits within your macronutrient goals. All the listed facts are based on

A Note about Alcohol

Although low-carb alcoholic beverages can certainly be enjoyed on a keto diet, including liquor and dry red wine in moderation, it won't do you any favors when it comes to fat loss and hormonal balance. In fact, alcohol induces inflammation and temporarily alters metabolism in a way that promotes fat storage.[21]

At 7 calories per gram, alcohol is almost as calorically dense as fat. And soon after consumption, your body immediately shifts to metabolizing the toxic substance—alcohol—and shuttles macronutrients off to storage as glycogen or body fat to burn up the alcohol as quickly as possible.[22] So, while your body handles the alcohol in your bloodstream, it delays burning the food you ate and fat on your body. Depending on how much or how frequently alcohol is consumed, it may be promoting fat storage—the complete opposite of what people reading this book are interested in.

Ketogenic diets also notoriously impair alcohol tolerance. If you decide to include alcohol in your diet occasionally, be careful not to overindulge.

Understanding a nutrition label on keto: is it a decent choice?

1
The Serving Size. Is that what you're really going to eat? The listed facts are based on this amount.

2
The total carbohydrate count. This number will help you decide if it will fit in your allowance.

3
Dietary fiber may be subtracted if you count net carbs. Much of the fiber in our diet is not absorbed.

4
Calories per serving. Calories will total all macronutrient values and help manage your overall intake.

5
Balance remaining macronutrients. Target adequate protein intake; align fat intake with your goals.

6
The ingredients. Listed in highest to lowest concentration. Check for problematic foods, such as allergens and food sensitivities. Sugars and starches trailing at the tail end of the list likely won't impact ketosis if overall carb count is low, but keep an eye out for sugars in disguise. If they are one of the primary ingredients: don't bother.

Nutrition Facts

8 servings per container

1	**Serving size**	**2/3 cup (55g)**

Amount per serving

4 **Calories** **230**

	% Daily Value*
5 **Total Fat** 8g	**10%**
Saturated Fat 1g	**5%**
Trans Fat 0g	
Cholesterol 0g	**0%**
Sodium 160mg	**7%**
2 **Total Carbohydrate** 37g	**13%**
3 Dietary Fiber 4g	**14%**
Total Sugars 12g	
Includes 10g Added Sugars	**20%**
5 **Protein** 3g	
Vitamin D 2mcg	10%
Calcium 260mg	20%
Iron 8mg	45%
Potassium 235mg	6%

*The % Daily Value (DV) tells you how much a nutrient in a serving of food contributes to a daily diet. 2,000 calories a day is used to general nutrition advice.

6 **INGREDIENTS:** enriched flour, corn syrup, sugar, soybean and palm oil, dextrose, high fructose corn syrup, fructose, glycerin, cocoa, polydextrose, modified corn starch, salt, dried cream, calcium carbonate, leavening, distilled monoglycerides, hydrogenated palm kernel oil, vanilla extract, xantham gum, natural and artificial flavor, yellow #5 lake, red #40 lake, caramel color, blue #2 lake, niacinamide, citric acid.

this amount. As an aside, the serving size is generally listed in two ways, volumetric and weight-based measurements. This can help you target the appropriate serving size using your preferred measurement device.

2. **Check total carbohydrates.** Now that you know the serving size, you can see whether this item fits within your overall daily macronutrient goals. As a rule of thumb (but not an unbreakable rule), you want this number to be less than 10 grams.

3. **Check the fiber.** If there are carbohydrates listed, dietary fiber is a great thing to see on a keto diet. Due to the low absorption of fiber, this nutrient has little impact on nutritional ketosis and overall calories. If you want to count net carbs—i.e., total carbs – fiber—this is one place to obtain the information.

4. **Check the calories per serving.** This number will tally all the energy provided by each macronutrient and help you balance your own energy requirements. It's a quick, easy tool to help you manage your intake. The carbs could be well within your range for ketosis, but if the calories will catapult you above your target, make your decision based on a different goal: losing body fat.

5. **Check the total fat and protein.** These numbers help you balance the remaining macronutrients. Are you shy of your protein goal and over on fat? Did you already meet your protein targets and have more room for fat? Remember, we are targeting adequate protein intake and aligning dietary fat consumption with our goals. These numbers will help you choose the foods that best align with your calculated macros.

6. **Check the ingredients list.** For some, this step might actually come before any of the others. If you are dealing with food allergies, are tackling the elimination step, or have food values that guide you to avoid certain ingredients or food additives, this is the place to check for them. In general, the fewer things listed, the better. It indicates less processing and more whole food ingredients. Ingredients are listed in highest to lowest concentration, which can also be insightful. Sugars and starches trailing in the tail end of the list are unlikely to affect ketosis, particularly if total carb count is low. If sugar and starches are the primary ingredients, you may want to pass and find better options.

On a cyclical keto diet, steps 2 and 5 change to focus on higher carb intake and lower fat intake on high-carb days.

Nutrient Databases

If you choose whole food ingredients—shopping the perimeter of the grocery store to purchase fresh produce rather than heading to the aisles to buy processed foods—you are going to find most of your food doesn't actually have a nutrition label. Rest assured, you can still find out the nutrient content. There are a plethora of databases available to determine the nutrient content of whole food ingredients. In many cases, this is the data food manufacturers use to develop their nutrition labels in the first place!

I recommend looking up nutrition information from online government databases, such as the USDA Nutrient Database or FoodData Central. These databases are compiled from evidence-based literature and undergo routine quality-control reviews, as opposed to the crowdsourced entries in other options. They also provide much more information regarding food than simple calorie and macronutrient values, including vitamin and mineral content and bioactive compounds. If you want to know the overall nutrient density of your meals, you can't beat these resources. See "Eating Strategies" (page 174) for information about tracking apps.

Measuring Your Food

When starting, you will do yourself a disservice if you don't measure your food and ingredients. We don't need laser-like precision, but we do need a reliable way to estimate our nutrient and calorie intake if we want results. Unfortunately, people are notoriously bad at estimating food amounts. Measuring can help you hone your estimation skills and ensure that what you think you are eating aligns with how much you actually eat. I strongly encourage you to use measuring tools, especially in the first phases of your diet.

Establishing a practice of measuring food can also be helpful if you run into a weight loss stall. You may be eating more than you think, and measuring can help you readjust.

Volume Measurements: Spoons, Cups, and Hands
Measuring spoons and cups can be useful instruments for measuring liquids, such as oils, broths, stocks, and nut milk when cooking. Use them when it makes sense. If you're using them to measure solid ingredients, don't overload the spoon or cup in heaping amounts; this can lead to excess. In the case of high-fat ingredients, such as nut butter, that can add up to hundreds of extra calories.

When not using a kitchen scale, this is the next best option for gauging appropriate serving sizes and monitoring portion control.

The Hand Method: The Zimbabwe Hand Jive
Your hand can also serve as a measuring device for estimating food portions—and it's one you'll never leave home without.

Dr. Kazzim Mawji developed a hand-based portion control method for his diabetic patients who were unable to use a portion scale, count calories, or count carbohydrates when managing their nutrition.[23] Today, the Zimbabwe Hand Jive is used throughout the world in diabetes management and fitness circles alike, due to its ease and effectiveness. Your hands can act as personalized measuring devices: Larger individuals with larger hands will require larger portions, and the smaller hands of smaller individuals facilitate smaller portions.[24]

A Case for the Kitchen Scale

When it comes to fat loss, I wish women would replace their bathroom scales with kitchen scales. Here's why:

- **You will calibrate your serving sizes**. If you have never measured your portions before, a kitchen scale can you help you dial in realistic amounts. There is something about seeing your food tallied to a precise number on the scale that just makes things click. The visual difference between one and two servings can be hard to differentiate by eyeballing alone, especially in calorie-dense foods such as fats and oils.

- **Volume measurements don't make sense for solid foods**. Unless you chop, dice, or purée ingredients, you will not be able to measure most solid foods in cups or spoon sizes. And would you want to? Imagine having a beautifully seared steak, but rather than diving in to enjoy it, you chopped it into tiny tidbits to stuff into a measuring cup first.

- **You can easily use unique serving sizes**. Using a kitchen scale also gives you the opportunity to work outside the confines of predefined serving sizes and volume measurements to tailor your actual intake with the nutrition data available. There is a considerable amount of variability between produce sizes. You will rarely get cuts of meat or pieces of fruit the same exact size. Placing your food on the scale gives you a more realistic idea of how much you eat and, in turn, a more effective way of accounting for your macros.

- **It's more efficient**. Using a scale to measure is much faster than using teaspoons and cups, and there is less to clean up in the end. Put your dish on the scale, tare it (reset it to zero), add your ingredient(s), and be on your way. Just one dish to clean! This can make meal-prep efforts easier as well.

If you aren't open to using a kitchen scale, rest assured, there are other options. This journey is about finding what is sustainable and realistic for you.

The concept is simple and can easily be applied to both the standard keto diet and alternative dieting methods discussed.

The palm of your hand shows the approximate size of a meat or fish portion for a meal, while the thickness of the meat is represented by the pinky.

> 1 palm = 1 portion of protein (meat, fish) = approximately 3 to 4 ounces (85 to 115 g)

Both hands cupped together represent a portion of low-carb vegetables or low-sugar fruit.

> 2 cupped hands = 1 portion of veggies or fruit = approximately 1 ounce (28 g)

Highly concentrated fats, such as oils and animal fats, can be measured with the thumb. One thumb represents about a tablespoon, while one thumbnail is approximately a teaspoon.

Helping Hands

Use this "handy" chart to visualize approximately sized portions for meals, snacks, and recipes (examples are provided for each corresponding measurement).

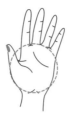

Palm ≈ 3-4 ounces
(Meat, fish & poultry.)

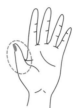

Thumb ≈ 1-2 tablespoons
(Concentrated fats and oils - salad dressing, sour cream, cream cheese & almond butter.)

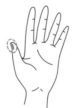

Thumbnail ≈ 1 teaspoon
(Concentrated fats and oils - salad dressing, sour cream, cream cheese & almond butter.)

Fist ≈ 1 cup
(Soups, casseroles, vegetables, fruits, and also starches and grains during high carb meals.)

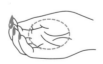

One cupped hand ≈ ½ cup
(Nuts, seeds & dairy.)

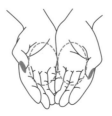

Two cupped hands ≈ 1 ounce
(Low carb vegetables & low sugar fruit.)

1 thumb = 1 tablespoon (weight varies) of concentrated fat (oils and fats)

1 thumbnail = 1 teaspoon of concentrated fat (oils and fats)

To measure other high-fat ingredients, such as nuts, seeds, and dairy, a portion fits in one cupped hand.

1 cupped hand = 1 portion of high-fat food (nuts, seeds, dairy)

During high-carb meals, one closed fist represents the size of a standard carbohydrate portion.

1 closed fist = 1 portion of carbs (grains and starches)[25]

How to Build a Keto Meal

We build our meals similarly to how we set our macros: protein first, carbs next, then fill in the remainder with fat. Building meals this way directly aligns our meals with our macros, helping achieve balance throughout the day, rather than scrambling to find appropriate foods.

1. **Choose a protein source:** meat, fish, or a vegetarian option.
2. **Layer in your carbohydrates:** vegetable, fruit, and/or spices.
3. **Fill the energy gap with fats:** oils, fats, nuts, seeds, or dairy.

This may sound overly simplistic, but it's a truly effective way to develop nutrient-dense meals that align with your individual goals. The combinations and options are endless. Simply adjust portions to coincide with your macros and meal frequency.

Working backward from the daily protein goal can give you a good starting point. For a reasonable per-meal protein goal, simply divide your daily protein target by the number of meals you plan to eat. For example, if you have a daily protein goal of 90 grams and plan to eat three meals, eating 30 grams of protein per meal can help you reach that target.

EXAMPLES OF A KETO MEAL STRUCTURE		
Protein	**Carbs**	**Fat**
Pork tenderloin	Cauliflower, cumin	Ghee, pine nuts
Chicken breast	Chayote squash, broth	Butter, heavy cream
Skirt steak	Bell pepper, onion, garlic	Olive oil
Ground beef	Zucchini, tomato	Cheese

How to Build a Keto Meal

Step 1
Choose a
protein source

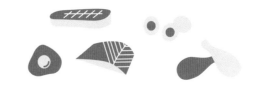

Step 2
Layer in
carbohydrates

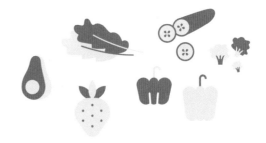

Step 3
Fill energy gap with fats
and oils (if needed)

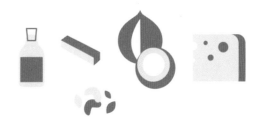

High Intensity Workouts
or Carb Cycling?
Slow digesting starches on
CKD days balanced with
lower fat intake, quick
digesting pre-workout carbs

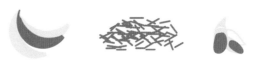

The same can be done with carbohydrates. Though you certainly don't have to eat up to 50 grams of carbs per day, divvying up the standard carb limit across your daily meals can help keep you within your limit throughout the day. If you have a maximum carb intake of 50 grams per day and plan to eat three meals, that allows room for up to 16 grams of carbohydrates (including fiber) per meal. Many dieters find they fall well below this number, which is perfectly fine; it's a limit, not a target, and everyone's carbohydrate tolerance differs.

Finally, with our fat macro, we can do something similar. However, unless your protein and carb sources provided zero fat content, we will also need to account for the fat supplied there. If you plan to eat a fatty cut of meat and avocado, then those sources provide a good amount of fat; there may not be a large energy gap to fill in with additional fats. When choosing lean meats and low-fat sources of carbohydrates, there will be more room for the extra fats. Also, remember some high-fat sources provide carbohydrates as well, namely nuts, seeds, and dairy. When using those as a fat source, balance that with your carbohydrate limit.

Eating Strategies: Tracking, Planning, and Intuitive Eating

When it comes to tallying calories and macros, there are tools to help you stay balanced and on track. Accounting for your intake with apps or something as simple as pen and paper can help you stay in tune with your daily meals and macros and help you adjust as needed. Many women feel empowered by tracking their intake, though not everyone gets that warm, fuzzy feeling about collecting the data behind their nourishment—and that's okay.

We will discuss three strategies that can help you work toward your goals. You may naturally gravitate toward hard data, metrics, and planning; you may prefer to live in the moment, be more spontaneous, and trust your instincts and feelings.

Let me ask you a simple question: How do you feel about spreadsheets? Your answer may be "How did you know?! I live for spreadsheets. I always have Excel open when I'm at my computer." If so, then you may very well be the data-loving planner who thrives on tracking your food intake with software or even your own system.

If, however, simply uttering the word "spreadsheet" leaves a particularly bad taste in your mouth, the practice of meticulously tracking your macros may not appeal to you. Although it's important to have a sensible estimate of your intake, getting too caught up in your diet minutiae may prove more stressful than anything.

Neither is right or wrong. Everyone has different modes of operation, backgrounds, and ways of thinking about their food.

Tracking Your Meals

Tracking your meals can help you keep track of your macros throughout the day. This can be done using websites, apps on your phone, or food journals. During the beginning phases, I find value in recording meals in a food journal to give space for thoughts, feelings, and personal insight. You can look up nutritional information on labels and databases, write down pertinent information about your food, and learn massive amounts as you go.

Looking up ingredients one by one in a nutrient database is not always the most convenient way of tracking. Phone and web-based apps can make it easier; they offer a convenient way to track meals and macros, pulling nutrition data from various sources and tallying nutrient information as you add ingredients. Some even provide bar-code scanners to pull up the data automatically. When choosing an app, use one that sources high-quality data, such as from a government database, rather than crowdsourced information. The Cronometer app is a favorite for this purpose; MyFitnessPal and Lose It! are also popular options.

Meal Planning

If the idea of winging your meals throughout the day incites panic and anxiety, consider meal planning based on your macro goals. Map out your meals ahead of time to ensure they coincide with your goals, create shopping lists based on the ingredients needed, and stick with your game plan for the week. Or do this on a smaller scale, outlining meals the day before.

One of the best resources for meal planning will be your food journal or log in your app. You can look back on previous entries, find meals you enjoyed or days that aligned with your macros particularly well, then re-cycle through them as you see fit. If something is working for you, you don't need to reinvent the wheel. Getting a wide variety of foods into your diet is vital for optimizing the nutrient density of it, but there is absolutely nothing wrong with having go-to meals, repeating what you ate during a previous week, or eating leftovers.

Intuitive Eating

After reading an entire book filled with diet details, you might be puzzled to see an intuitive eating suggestion. Rather than placing emphasis on calories and macros, intuitive eating is all about connecting with your body and listening to its cues for nourishment. Here are some ways to think about intuitive eating practices:

· Eat when your body sends hunger signals; stop when you feel full.
· Dedicate time to eat your meal and focus on the food, rather than mindlessly taking in nourishment while driving, working, or watching television.
· Get in tune with things that trigger emotional eating.
· Forgive yourself when things don't go as planned.
· Ditch the "good" food, "bad" food mind-set.

- Keep a food journal that gauges your feelings, moods, and thoughts before and after a meal, versus one exclusively focused on nutrient data.
- Most importantly, be flexible with your diet.

It's not about restricting; it's about finding foods that work the best with your body and being mindful of your eating. If keto provides the foods you find enjoyable and sustainable, trusting your body to guide your food choices can be just as powerful, if not more so, than any diet-tracking app on the market.

So, now that you know some great keto-compatible foods and how to incorporate them into meals to align with your macros, you are almost ready to get started. There's just one more thing on our agenda: supplements for optimal success.

12

Supplements for Optimal Success

L et's briefly review supplements that will help you feel your best and optimize your success on the keto diet. Although I recommend striving to obtain nutrient support from your diet, there are times when supplementation can be helpful. This chapter will help you target areas that may require supplementation on keto, support hormonal balance, and address common deficiencies that women experience.

Avoiding "Keto Flu"

"Keto flu" is the electrolyte imbalance that commonly occurs after switching to a keto diet. Symptoms can feel similar to the flu: shakiness, dizziness, nausea, headaches, diarrhea, and cramps. They're due to a change in your body's sodium metabolism. When something changes in your body, your body immediately starts working to restore balance. Our starting point is typically a standard Western diet full of high-sodium and low-potassium foods, which causes the kidneys to retain excess sodium.[1]

As you shift into the metabolic state of ketosis, insulin levels drop. This triggers the body to release sodium.[2] Your kidneys begin to excrete it, along with buckets of water. Your sodium level transitions from excess to depleted, which triggers another balancing mechanism, which causes potassium excretion to follow suit. As water is released, other water-soluble vitamins and minerals can also be flushed out. This process describes what is known as "the natriuresis of fasting" resulting from carb restriction.[3]

Luckily, simply replenishing sodium and potassium can resolve the issue. You can prevent keto flu altogether by consuming adequate amounts of both. As you continue with keto, your body will adapt, though electrolyte management will still be a priority.

Sodium

Due to the carbohydrate restriction on a standard keto diet, you require sodium. The easiest way to get adequate amounts is by including salt in your diet. Liberally salt your food and enjoy broths, stocks, and even bouillon (though they many contain small amounts of sugar and food additives). Salty brines, such as pickle juice, are also a keto favorite. Additionally, electrolyte supplements that provide salt can be used as long as they don't also contain carbohydrates.

Signs of low sodium include fatigue, low energy, headache, nausea, vomiting, confusion, irritability, and lightheadedness.

The current adequate intake (AI), or approximate nutrient needs, for sodium are set to cover basic sodium sweat losses; however, it does not apply to individuals who lose large volumes of sodium.[4] That includes athletes who release large amounts of sodium in sweat and keto dieters dumping sodium via natriuresis. The AI for most women is 1.5 grams of sodium daily and a tolerable upper intake level of 2.3 grams,[5] but we need more than that. Instead, aim for 4 to 5 grams of sodium per day, or more depending on your physical activity. Also, listen to the cues your body is sending if you prefer not to measure and track; if you are feeling woozy after starting keto, it might be time to sip some broth.

Potassium

Once you correct your sodium levels, potassium will adjust as long as you replenish it. Simply increasing dietary potassium intake is a practical and effective approach to bringing potassium to adequate levels without any supplementation. In most scenarios, it is also preferable. Potassium plays a role in electrolyte balance and many critical biological processes.

Low potassium symptoms include constipation, tiredness, muscle weakness, and irregular heart rate.

Potassium-rich keto-compatible foods include avocados, fish, meat, dark leafy greens, bone broth, nuts, mushrooms, and dairy as well as low-sodium salt products, such as NoSalt or Lite Salt, which often partially replace sodium with potassium. Recommended daily potassium intake is as follows:

- Adult women: 4,700 milligrams
- Pregnant women: 4,700 milligrams
- Breastfeeding women: 5,100 milligrams
- Tolerable upper intake Level: not set for healthy adults[6]

On average, women in the United States get only 2,320 milligrams of potassium from food per day, less than half that recommended![7]

If you are unable to source appropriate potassium from your diet, consider supplementation. Potassium supplements can be found in many multivitamin forms and also individually, listed as potassium chloride, potassium citrate, potassium phosphate, potassium aspartate, potassium bicarbonate, and potassium gluconate in the ingredients.[8]

However, potassium supplementation is not for everyone. Excess potassium levels can be dangerous and may lead to hyperkalemia; women with a history of diabetes, renal insufficiency, or heart failure are at high risk for this. Additionally, potassium supplements are contraindicated with blood-pressure medications and some potassium-sparing diuretics. Work with your doctor for individual guidance.

Common Nutrient Deficiencies for Women

In addition to the lower levels of sodium and potassium that result from the start of a keto diet, there are some nutrient deficiencies particularly common among women. Let's address them.

Magnesium

Magnesium is required for cellular uptake of potassium. Simply increasing magnesium will help your body use more of the potassium it takes in. As you work to replenish potassium levels, magnesium supplementation is recommended.

The benefits of magnesium are vast, especially for women. Magnesium supports stress management and thyroid health and aids sleep, hormone production, and bone health. If you experience constipation after changing to a keto diet, magnesium can be an effective remedy. It is known for its calming, relaxing effects, which can help you get a good night's sleep, manage stress, and balance cortisol levels.[9] The relaxing effects can help you combat migraines and tension headaches if they should arise as well.[10]

Signs of low magnesium include headaches, migraines, cramps (including menstrual cramps), constipation, anxiety, irritability, depression, mood disorders, PMS, fatigue, and difficulty sleeping.

Foods highest in magnesium are often those high in fiber. Good keto-compatible dietary sources of magnesium include a range of vegetables (such as leafy greens and broccoli), seaweed, nuts, seeds, avocado, fatty fish, tofu, coffee, dairy, meats, and dark chocolate (in moderation). Hard water, or water with high mineral content, can also be a source of magnesium. At higher-carb meals, grains and legumes provide magnesium sources as well. Recommended daily magnesium intake is:

- Adult women: 310 to 320 milligrams
- Pregnant women: 350 to 360 milligrams
- Breastfeeding women: 310 to 320 milligrams
- Tolerable upper intake level: 350 milligrams[11]

Magnesium oxide is the most common form of magnesium found in supplements, but it's also notorious for having the lowest bioavailability, mainly acting as a laxative. Magnesium sulfate also has low bioavailability but can be soothing to sore muscles soaked in a bath—Epsom salts contain it. Absorption of magnesium supplements varies; however, magnesium salts are more completely absorbed in the gut, as they dissolve well in liquid.[12] Forms of magnesium with the best absorption include magnesium citrate, magnesium glycinate, magnesium threonate, magnesium malate, and magnesium taurate.[13]

Include magnesium-rich foods in your diet, but consider supplementing your daily routine if you experience symptoms of low magnesium. Magnesium supplementation can be particularly helpful as you work to correct keto-flu symptoms related to low potassium.

Iron
Women lose iron regularly during menstrual bleeds. If we don't replenish lost iron in the interim, we run the risk of becoming deficient, and, over time, anemia can develop. Women with heavy flows and vegetarians are at particularly high risk.

Iron is needed to make certain hormones, including thyroid hormone synthesis. When iron levels are low, thyroid hormone production dips. So, on top of feeling lousy, your metabolic rate can drop as well. Getting adequate iron in the diet or via supplementation can help boost levels back to normal.

Keto-compatible dietary sources of iron include meat, seafood, poultry, nuts, and spinach, though the plant-based sources are not absorbed as well.

Women who are still menstruating require a higher daily iron intake than postmenopausal women due to regular blood loss. Pregnant women require even more as a result of increased blood volume during pregnancy. Vegetarian women require approximately double the amount of iron due to the poor absorption of plant-based iron.[14] Recommended daily iron intake is:

- Women under 50 years: 18 milligrams
- Women over 50 years: 8 milligrams
- Pregnant women: 27 milligrams

- Breastfeeding women: 9 milligrams
- Vegetarian women: double the amount for the relevant category
- Tolerable upper intake limit: 45 milligrams[15]

Iron is available in many daily multivitamins designed for women and as a supplement of its own. There are generally two types of iron used in the supplements: ferric and ferrous iron salts. Ferrous iron is the more bioavailable of the two, so look for ferrous sulfate or ferrous gluconate if you require supplementation.[16]

Vitamin D

Vitamin D is vital for fat loss, hormonal health, immune system health, bone health, and mood. It has many critical roles in the body, yet many of us struggle to get enough.

Very few foods naturally provide vitamin D, but the body makes vitamin D when directly exposed to the sun. If you live in a sunny area 365 days a year and you head outdoors once a day, chances are you won't need a supplement. But if you live in an area where cloudy days are abundant, vitamin D supplementation may be warranted.

Food sources include fatty fish, beef liver, egg yolk, mushrooms, and vitamin D–fortified dairy products.[17]

If you can, make a conscious effort to get outdoors and soak up the rays. But that's not always possible. Perhaps it's winter, and you haven't seen the sun in months. Maybe you live in a beautiful sunny area but are trapped inside at work all day. Or perhaps you work the night shift and sleep while the sun is out. It happens. Recommended daily vitamin D intake is:

- Women under 70 years: 600 IU
- Women over 70 require: 800 IU
- Tolerable upper intake limit: 4,000 IU[18]

There are two forms of vitamin D supplements on the market: D_2 (ergocalciferol) and D_3 (cholecalciferol); both are absorbed well and increase blood levels of vitamin D.[19] However, some studies show that vitamin D_3 is a more potent form of the supplement, with more significant increases to vitamin D blood levels.[20]

Calcium

Calcium is incredibly important for women, yet many of us don't get nearly enough from the foods we eat. Women are at high risk for bone density loss as we age, making calcium intake critical to supporting bone health and preventing osteoporosis. You need calcium throughout your life but require even more as you get older.

Dairy can be an excellent source of calcium for women on a keto diet, but for the dairy-free dieter, it can be difficult to obtain adequate amounts. Some dark leafy greens, such as spinach, provide calcium, but it is poorly absorbed due to the oxalate content. Recommended daily calcium intake IS:

- Women under 50 years: 1,000 milligrams
- Women over 50 years: 1,200 milligrams
- Tolerable upper intake limit: 2,500 milligrams[21]

If your diet limits your calcium intake, consider supplementing. Look for calcium citrate, as it is more easily absorbed than the alternative calcium carbonate supplements.[22]

Iodine

There is a lot of controversy surrounding iodine, particularly when it comes to women's thyroid health. Iodine is imperative for healthy thyroid function. It is one of the building blocks of your thyroid hormones, and without adequate iodine, your thyroid is unable to produce sufficient levels of its hormones. This can lead to lower thyroid levels and contribute to hypothyroidism. However, excess intake, particularly in the absence of selenium, may cause thyroid dysfunction.[23] Recommended daily iodine intake is:

- Adult women: 150 micrograms
- Pregnant women: 220 micrograms
- Breastfeeding women: 290 micrograms
- Tolerable upper intake limit: 1,100 micrograms[24]

Dietary sources of iodine include iodized salt (though not all salts are iodized), dairy, eggs, fish, and other seafood. Deficiencies can develop with reduced salt intake, avoidance of iodized salt, and diets lacking dairy, eggs, and seafood. Additionally, goitrogenic foods, including soy and cruciferous vegetables, can interfere with the way the body uses iodine and may be problematic for women with low thyroid levels.

For thyroid health, consider supplementing iodine if you are unable to obtain appropriate amounts from food sources. The American Thyroid Association advises against the ingestion of iodine supplements over 500 micrograms daily.[25] However, if you have an autoimmune thyroid disease, such as Hashimoto's, consult your health care provider before increasing iodine intake or supplementing, as increased iodine may be contraindicated.

Selenium supplementation is also beneficial for thyroid support.[26]

Detox: Support Your Liver

I also recommend detoxification support. I'm not suggesting a detox diet of special juices and elixirs; I'm talking about your liver, your own personal detoxification system. The detoxification pathways in your liver require specific nutrients to support the reactions. A diet with high-quality protein—a complete amino acid profile—and a variety of nonstarchy veggies and low-sugar fruits will get you off to a good start. Consider a glutathione or N-acetyl cysteine (NAC) supplement as well.

As you lose body fat, stored hormones, toxins, and pollutants are released. As a result, your liver goes to town metabolizing them to release from your body. Without adequate nutritional support, they can't be appropriately processed, and they stay in the body. This negatively affects hormonal balance and can affect weight loss efforts as well. Glutathione can help neutralize toxins in the liver, and NAC serves to replenish glutathione levels.

Support your liver during periods of fat loss with a glutathione or NAC supplement. Oral supplements of glutathione can be degraded in the intestine prior to absorption, and N-acetyl cysteine can be a more effective way to boost glutathione levels.

Gut Support & Repair

To support a healthy balance of good bacteria in our gut (see page 91), it is essential to include prebiotics and probiotics in our diet and supplement routine.

Prebiotics are food for the good bacteria—and that means fiber. Keto-compatible prebiotic food sources include vegetables such as asparagus, eggplant, endive, artichoke, onion, garlic, cabbage, and radish; some dairy products, such as kefir and yogurt; and high-fiber seeds, such as flax, chia, and hemp.

Probiotics, on the other hand, *are* the good bacteria! By regularly replenishing the good guys, we provide a diverse microbiome and ensure the pathogenic bad guys do not outcompete for the territory. Fermented foods can provide an excellent source of probiotics in our diet.

You can easily prepare fermented foods at home or purchase them at the grocery store; when shopping for foods containing healthy bacteria, look for the words "live cultures" on the container and choose raw, unpasteurized options when available. Note that heat from cooking will destroy the bacteria. An additional keto-related benefit of the fermentation process is the carbohydrate content is reduced as the bacteria work to ferment the carbs.

Keto-compatible fermented foods include aged cheese, cottage cheese, fermented meats and fish, fermented vegetables (including sauerkraut and kimchi), kefir (plain, unsweetened), kombucha (plain, unsweetened), cultured creams (including sour cream and crème fraîche), and yogurt (plain, unsweetened).

Alternately, take prebiotic and probiotic supplements. If you have difficulty incorporating fiber-rich and fermented foods into your daily regimen, consider supplementation to support a healthy gut. Commercially available prebiotic supplements include galactooligosaccharides (GOS), fructooligosaccharides (FOS), and lactulose.

To aid in gut repair from inflammation, damaged tissue, and leaky gut (see page 90), consider taking an L-glutamine supplement. It is the preferred food source of cells in the small intestine and can help restore the barrier that reduces intestinal permeability.

Supplements to Consider

Calcium	Prebiotics
Glutathione	Probiotics
Iodine	Protein
Iron	Selenium
L-glutamine	Sodium
Magnesium	Vitamin D
Potassium	

Protein: Alternative Sources

Dietary sources of protein are more readily absorbed, are more sating, and offer higher nutrient density than supplements. Though protein shakes and powders can be enjoyed as an ingredient in smoothies, puddings and baked goods, and even by themselves, I tucked them away in the supplement chapter to emphasize that they are supplements, not meal replacements.

There are hundreds of protein powders on the market. Some contain dairy or artificial ingredients some dieters avoid, so look at the nutrition label and ingredients list to determine whether something is an acceptable choice for keto and your food values.

Not all protein supplements are complete proteins. Animal-based protein powders, such as whey, casein, and egg white, contain all essential amino acids, but plant-based protein powders lack the full range. Plant-based mixes also tend to be higher in carbohydrates. Collagen is an exception to the rule as an animal-based protein source that is not a complete protein.

If you supplement your diet with protein powders, pick high-quality ingredients that align with your personal needs. As new brands and products hit the market every day, with different tastes, textures, and components, finding one you love can mean a bit of trial and error. To narrow your search, I encourage you to read reviews and visit sites that investigate the quality and label claims via third-party testing—Labdoor (labdoor.com), for example.

Where Do You Go from Here?

Now that you have all the tools to get started, it's time to take the plunge. Remember, there is no such thing as perfect, so don't let that keep you from taking action. Whether you start small, adding a few keto-compatible foods to your next grocery list, or you dive in head first, what matters is that you're working toward your goal.

Take imperfect action. Celebrate the small wins. Be mindful and present. Be flexible but realistic. Listen to your body. Don't compare your progress to others'. Do what works best for you, not for someone else. Take one day at a time, knowing each small step will take you closer to your goal.

And while you're at it, snap a photo or record a video of yourself to look back on. You'll thank me later.

Imperfect action is better than perfect inaction.

— *Harry S. Truman*

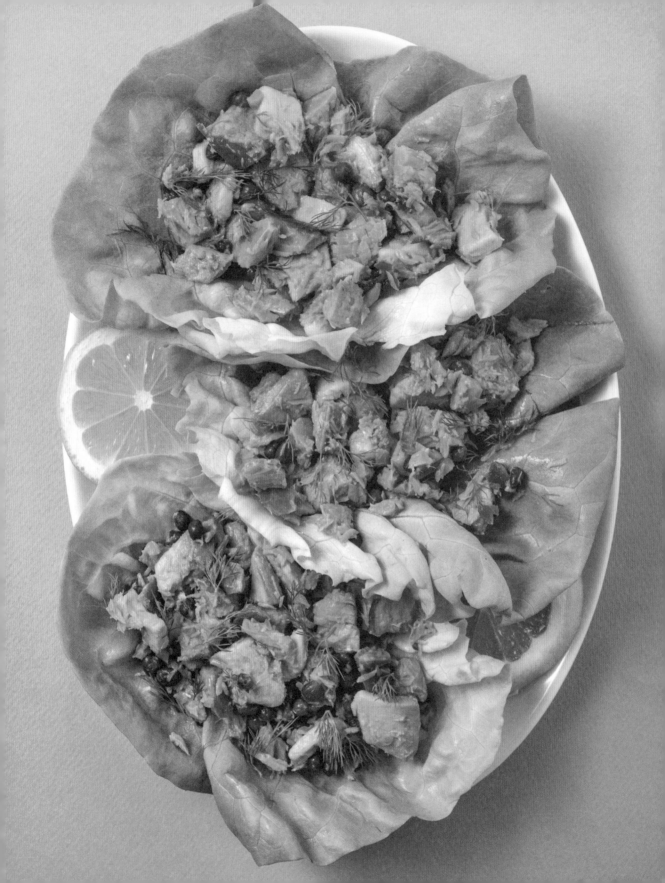

RECIPES

In chapter 11, you learned how to build easy keto meals by combining a protein source of your choice, low carb veggies or fruit, and healthful fats. Following that template will set you up for eating simple, delicious meals that support your goals and food preferences without overcomplicating things. It really is that easy!

I wholeheartedly believe that the best thing you can do to improve your health is to start cooking at home. When you're first starting out with new dietary changes, having examples of what types of meals to eat can be extremely beneficial. And if you are just learning to cook, having step-by-step instructions on what to do with all of your healthy ingredients can be a lifesaver!

The recipes in this book are designed to do just that—get you cooking with keto-compatible ingredients! Following the meal building template, I've developed a variety of recipes that range from no-cook meals to more elaborate cooking projects, complete with detailed macronutrient data. These dishes are designed to be flexible, allowing you to tailor them to meet your personal preferences. Don't like the main protein? Swap it out for another! Don't have an ingredient on hand? Use what's in your fridge! I encourage you to adapt these recipes to suit your individual needs, whether it is for taste, potential allergens, or just to get creative and experiment. Enjoy!

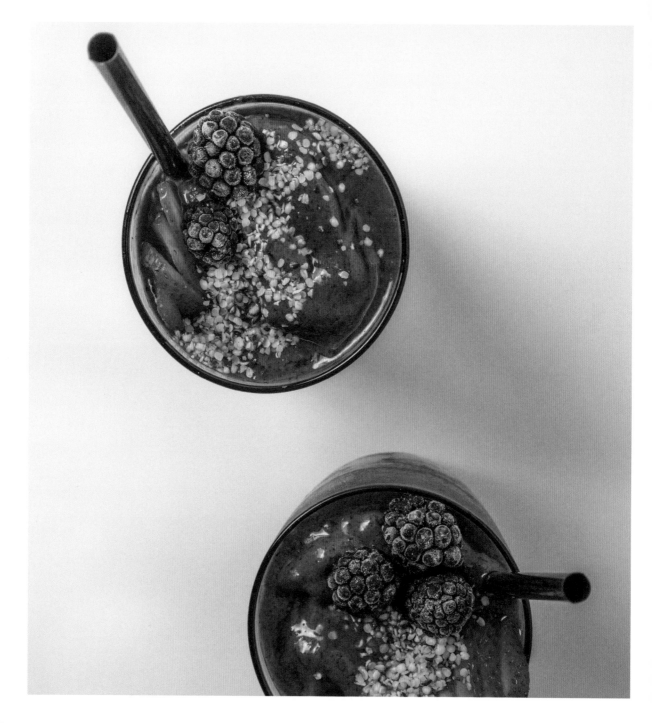

NUTRITION FACTS: **Full Recipe:** 328 calories, 14 g fat, total carbs 23.2 g, 12.9 g fiber (10.28 g net carbs), 30.6 g protein
Per Serving: 164 calories, 7 g fat, total carbs 11.6 g, 6.5 g fiber (5.14 g net carbs), 15.3 g protein

Keto Smoothie

YIELD: 2 servings
SERVING SIZE: 1 smoothie (half of the recipe)

PREP TIME: 5 minutes
TOTAL TIME: 5 minutes

Smoothies can be a great way to pack in nutrient-dense ingredients, but they are often full of sugar and carbohydrates. Choosing low sugar fruits, fibrous veggies, and unsweetened liquids will help you keep carbs low. Feel free to experiment!

INGREDIENTS:

½ avocado

1 cup (30 g) spinach

1 cup (144 g) fresh or frozen blackberries

1 cup (235 ml) unsweetened, plain almond milk

2 cups (217 g) ice

1 scoop (30 g) low-carb protein powder such as Dymatize ISO 100 (optional)

INSTRUCTIONS:

1. Add ingredients to blender and close lid.

2. Pulse until ingredients are smoothly blended and serve.

NOTE: Carbohydrate content and ingredients vary dramatically between brands and product lines of protein powder. Be sure to read the ingredients and nutrition facts to ensure the protein powder aligns with your needs and goals. Alternatively, feel free to skip the protein powder altogether!

DIY Granola Bars

YIELD: 12 servings (12 bars)
SERVING SIZE: 1 bar

PREP TIME: 15 minutes
COOK TIME: 35 minutes

TOTAL TIME: 50 minutes

These DIY granola bars are the perfect on-the-go breakfast!

SPECIAL DIET CONSIDERATIONS: This recipe contains nuts and eggs.

INGREDIENTS:

2 ounces (55 g) hulled hemp seeds (hemp hearts)

2 ounces (55 g) sliced almonds

1 ounce (28 g) chopped almonds

2 ounces (55 g) pumpkin seeds (pepitas)

2 ounces (55 g) flaxseed meal

1 ounce (28 g) sesame seeds

2 egg whites

1 whole egg

1 tablespoon (16 g) unsweet-ened almond butter or nut butter of your choice

½ teaspoon vanilla extract

½ teaspoon ground cinnamon

INSTRUCTIONS:

1. Preheat oven to 300°F (150°C or gas mark 2). Line an 11 × 7-inch (28 × 18 cm) brownie pan or casserole dish with parchment paper.

2. Combine hemp seeds, almonds, pumpkin seeds, flaxseed meal, and sesame seeds in a large bowl.

3. In a separate large bowl, whisk egg whites until soft peaks form. Stir in the whole egg, nut butter, vanilla, and cinnamon.

4. Add seed and nut mixture and thoroughly combine.

5. Transfer mixture to parchment paper–lined pan and press into an even layer.

6. Bake for 25 to 35 minutes or until golden brown.

7. Remove from oven and transfer the granola in parchment to a cooling rack. Cut into 12 pieces, approximately 1½ × 3½ inches (4 × 9 cm) each. Store in an airtight container or zipper lock bag in the refrigerator until ready to serve.

NOTE: Dark chocolate chips, cacao nibs, or a low-carb sweetener of your choice can be added to sweeten the bars if you desire.

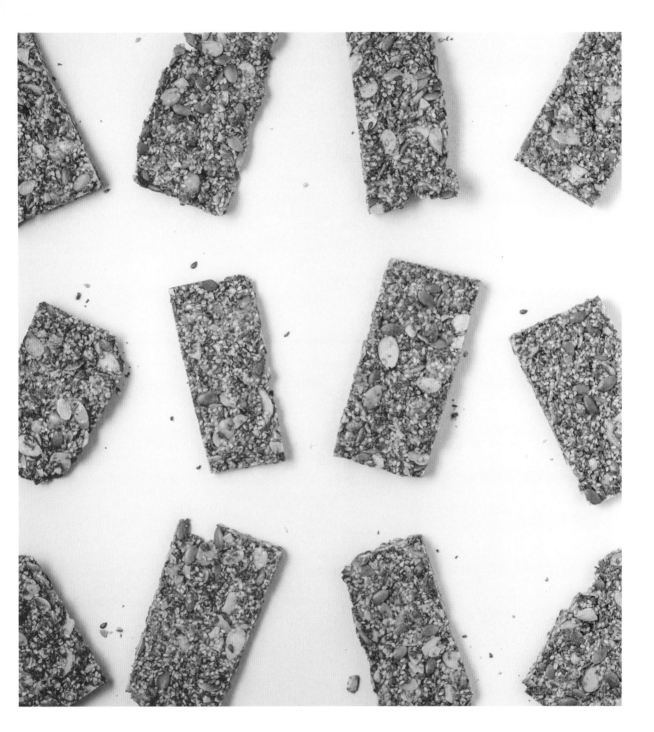

NUTRITION FACTS: **Full Recipe:** 1,784 calories, 144 g fat, 61.8 g total carbs, 39.6 g fiber (22.2 g net carbs), 88.6 g protein
Per Granola Bar: 149 calories, 12 g fat, 5.2 g total carbs, 3.3 g fiber (1.9 g net carbs), 7.4 g protein

Keto Oatmeal

YIELD: 1 serving
SERVING SIZE: 1 recipe

PREP TIME: 5 minutes
COOK TIME: 5 minutes

TOTAL TIME: 10 minutes

If the idea of giving up a warm bowl of oatmeal in the name of keto is keeping you up at night, fear not! With a little culinary creativity, we can re-create the breakfast classic with keto-compatible ingredients. Best of all, this oatmeal is loaded with magnesium and omega-3 fatty acids.

INGREDIENTS:

¼ cup (36 g) hulled hemp seeds (hemp hearts)

1 tablespoon (7 g) coconut flour

1 tablespoon (7 g) flaxseed meal

1 tablespoon (13 g) chia seeds

¼ cup (60 ml) plain, unsweetened coconut, almond, macadamia, or hemp milk

1 tablespoon (15 ml) water

½ teaspoon ground cinnamon

½ teaspoon vanilla extract

erythritol, monk fruit, or stevia sweetener to taste (optional, if tolerated)

INSTRUCTIONS:

1. Combine hemp seeds, coconut flour, flaxseed meal, chia seeds, milk, and 1 tablespoon (15 ml) of water in a small saucepan.

2. Bring to a boil and then reduce to a simmer over medium-low heat until thickened to desired consistency.

3. Stir in cinnamon and vanilla extract. Stir in a small amount of sweetener, if using, to taste.

4. Serve immediately or store in airtight glass container in the refrigerator for up to 3 days to easily reheat.

NOTE: The recipe is a great oatmeal base. You can adjust the ingredients and add toppings of your choice to customize the flavor profile and add variety! It's also an easy make-ahead meal—simply mix in a small amount of water and reheat on the stovetop or in the microwave.

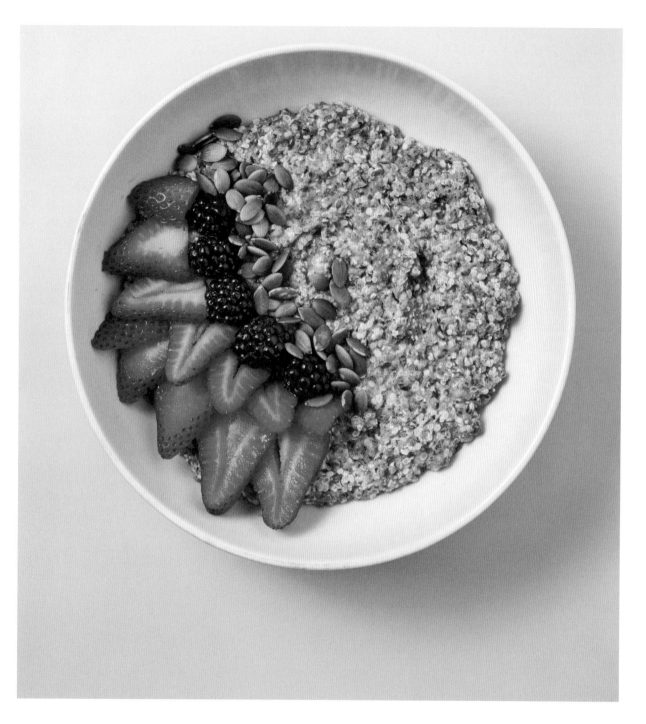

NUTRITION FACTS: **Full Recipe:** 355.7 calories, 27.2 g fat, 15.4 g total carbs, 10.1 g fiber (5.23 g net carbs), 17 g protein.

Coconut Yogurt

YIELD: 6 servings
SERVING SIZE: 4 ounces (115 g)
PREP TIME: 5 minutes

COOK TIME: 10 minutes
INCUBATION TIME: 24 hours
TOTAL TIME: 24 hours 15 minutes

Fermented foods are so much fun to prepare. It's like a delicious, decadent science project in your kitchen! Yogurts, such as this one made from coconut milk, have the additional benefit of acting as a probiotic. This can help your gut heal gastrointestinal issues and restore hormonal balance. If you have a particular probiotic strain that you take for health purposes, consider adding it to your yogurt creation in addition to the yogurt starter cultures.

SPECIAL DIET CONSIDERATIONS: Replace the gelatin with agar agar to make this recipe vegetarian.

INGREDIENTS:

2 cans (13.5 ounces, or 382 g each) of coconut milk

1 tablespoon (17 g) gelatin

1 packet powdered yogurt starter

Optional toppings

berries

chopped nuts

seeds

INSTRUCTIONS:

1. Bring coconut milk and gelatin to a boil and then remove from heat and allow to cool down to 110°F (43°C). Use a thermometer to track the temperature.

2. Once the milk mixture has cooled to the desired temperature, mix in yogurt starter, taking care to use sterile utensils.

3. Transfer the mixture to a sterilized yogurt maker to incubate at 110°F to 115°F (43°C to 46°C). Alternatively, use sterile lidded canning jars to hold the coconut milk mixture and incubate at 110°F to 115°F (43°C to 46°C). When using this method, incubation at the desired temperature range can be achieved using a water bath heated to 110°F (43°C) with an immersion circulator tool (as used in sous vide cooking), though some find success simply incubating in the oven with the light turned on.

4. Incubate for 24 hours, then refrigerate. Store in the refrigerator for up to a week.

NOTE: If you prefer, you can replace yogurt starter with probiotic capsules to inoculate the yogurt. You will need probiotics that contain two essential species responsible for yogurt-making magic: *Lactobacillus delbrueckii* spp. *bulgaricus* and *Streptococcus thermophilus*.

NUTRITION FACTS:

Full Recipe: 1,363 calories, 132 g fat, 12 g total carbs, 0 g fiber (12 g net carbs), 23 g protein
Per Serving: 227 calories, 22 g fat, 2 g total carbs, 0 g fiber (2 g net carbs), 3.8 g protein

Eggs Benedict on Portobello

YIELD: 4 servings; ½ cup (115 ml) hollandaise
SERVING SIZE: 1 mushroom cap, 1 egg, ¼ of the ham, and 2 tablespoons (28 ml) hollandaise sauce

PREP TIME: 10 minutes
COOK TIME: 20 minutes
TOTAL TIME: 30 minutes

Skip the English muffins and give your Eggs Benedict a low carb base instead! Portobello mushrooms work perfectly as a bread replacement in this recipe, but feel free to get creative.

SPECIAL DIET CONSIDERATIONS: This recipe is not dairy-free because ghee is used in the hollandaise sauce. However, ghee (also known as clarified butter) contains no lactose or milk proteins, making it a relatively safe option for many with lactose intolerance and casein or whey sensitivities. However, trace amounts of lactose and milk proteins may be present in ghee; you may want to avoid this ingredient if you have or suspect dairy allergies.

INGREDIENTS:

Roasted Portobellos

4 portobello mushroom caps, stems removed

¼ teaspoon avocado oil or cooking oil of choice

Poached Eggs

1 tablespoon (15 ml) vinegar

4 eggs

Hollandaise Sauce

2 egg yolks

2 tablespoons (28 ml) lemon juice

1 tablespoon (15 ml) cold water

2 tablespoons (28 ml) melted ghee

1 to 4 tablespoons (15 to 60 ml) hot water

salt to taste

Eggs Benedict

8 ounces (225 g) uncured ham or Canadian bacon, thinly sliced

INSTRUCTIONS:

Roasted Portobellos

1. Preheat oven to 400°F (200°C or gas mark 6).

2. Spray or brush a thin coat of oil on portobello mushrooms. Place gill-side up on baking sheet and cook in oven for 10 minutes. Remove pan and carefully flip each mushroom. Add ham or Canadian bacon to pan and bake for an additional 5 minutes.

3. Keep warm until ready to serve.

Poached Eggs

1. Bring 1 inch (2.5 cm) of water to a simmer in a large saucepan or skillet over medium heat. Add vinegar to water.

2. Carefully crack eggs into individual ramekins, taking care not to break the yolks. Alternatively, work with one egg at a time.

3. Slowly pour one egg at a time into the simmering water, spaced away from the others, taking care not to break the yolks. Allow to cook for 3 to 4 minutes or until the white of the egg is thoroughly cooked and the yolk is still soft. Remove eggs with a slotted spoon and reserve until ready to construct Eggs Benedict.

(continued)

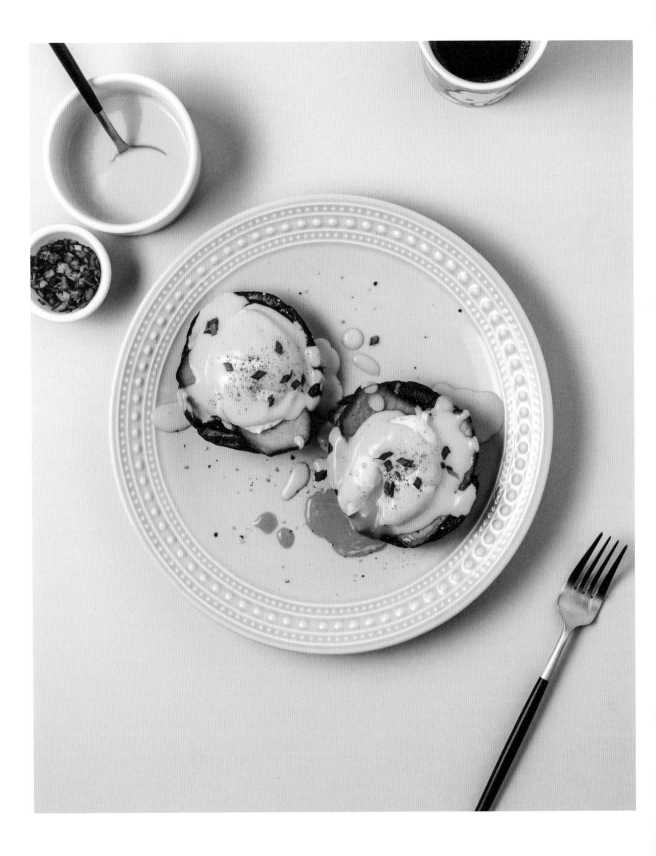

(continued)

Hollandaise Sauce

1. Heat a small saucepan filled with water over medium heat.

2. In an aluminum mixing bowl, whisk egg yolks, lemon juice, and cold water until mixture becomes frothy. Carefully place mixing bowl over the heated water in the saucepan and continue whisking.

3. Slowly drizzle in ghee, whisking continuously, until hollandaise sauce sets up.

4. If sauce becomes too thick, whisk in a small amount of hot water from the saucepan one tablespoon (28 ml) at a time until you reach desired consistency. Add salt to taste.

Eggs Benedict

Place a mushroom cap on a plate gill-side up and layer ham, egg, and two tablespoons (28 ml) of hollandaise sauce on top.

NOTE: This recipe also works well on top of other vegetables—steamed asparagus, sliced raw avocado, roasted eggplant, sliced tomatoes, you name it!

Poached eggs can be made ahead of time and placed in the refrigerator until ready to serve. Simply place in hot water for 20 to 30 seconds to reheat. I often make poached eggs as part of my weekly meal prep to use for in more labor-intensive meals like this one, on top of a bunless burger, in soups, or in veggie noodle pasta.

NUTRITION FACTS:

Eggs Benedict without Hollandaise Sauce
Full Recipe: 650 calories, 29 g fat, 18.4 g total carbs, 4.4 g fiber (14.08 g net carbs), 76.2 g protein
Per Serving: 162 calories, 7.3 g fat, 4.6 g total carbs, 1.1 g fiber (3.52 g net carbs), 19 g protein

Hollandaise Sauce
Full Recipe: 338 calories, 34 g fat, 3.3 g total carbs, 0.1 g fiber (3.2 g net carbs), 5.4 g protein
Per Serving: 84 calories, 8.6 g fat, 0.8 g total carbs, 0 g fiber (0.8 g net carbs), 1.4 g protein

Eggs Benedict with Hollandaise Sauce

Full Recipe: 988 calories, 63 g fat, 21.7 g total carbs, 4.5 g fiber (17.28 g net carbs), 81.6 g protein
Per Serving: 246 calories, 15.9 g fat, 5.3 g total carbs, 1.1 g fiber (4.32 g net carbs), 20.4 g protein

Savory Steamed Egg Custard

YIELD: 2 servings
SERVING SIZE: half of the recipe

PREP TIME: 5 minutes
COOK TIME: 8 minutes

TOTAL TIME: 13 minutes

Steamed eggs are delicate, creamy, and totally compatible with a standard low carb keto diet! This tender egg custard is a perfect light breakfast or side, but you can easily transform this dish into a substantial meal with various meat, seafood, or vegetable toppings.

INGREDIENTS:

4 large eggs

1 cup (235 ml) room temperature chicken broth or water

1 dash salt

2 teaspoons garlic-infused olive oil or sesame oil (optional)

⅛ teaspoon coconut aminos or soy sauce

1 tablespoon (3 g) minced chives

INSTRUCTIONS:

1. Pour 1 inch (2.5 cm) of water into the bottom of a large steamer pan with a fitted lid and set on stove burner. Place a fitted steamer rack above the water line, cover with the lid, and turn to high heat to produce steam.

2. In a small mixing bowl, gently stir eggs, chicken broth, and salt together, taking care not to whisk in air bubbles. Strain mixture through a fine mesh strainer into a large, pourable measuring cup.

3. Divide mixture between two small, heat-safe glass bowls, ramekins, or chawanmushi dishes and cover the tops tightly with foil or fitted lids. Carefully place each dish into the steamer rack, cover steamer with lid, and steam for 8 minutes or until the egg is just set.

4. Remove the dishes from the steamer and discard foil. Garnish with oil, coconut aminos, and chives. Serve immediately.

NOTE: Smaller dishes may require less time in the steamer, larger dishes more; the egg is ready when it is appears solid and jiggles in its container.

Feel free to experiment with various toppings; shrimp, chicken, mushrooms, bell pepper, or hot sauce would all be fantastic additions!

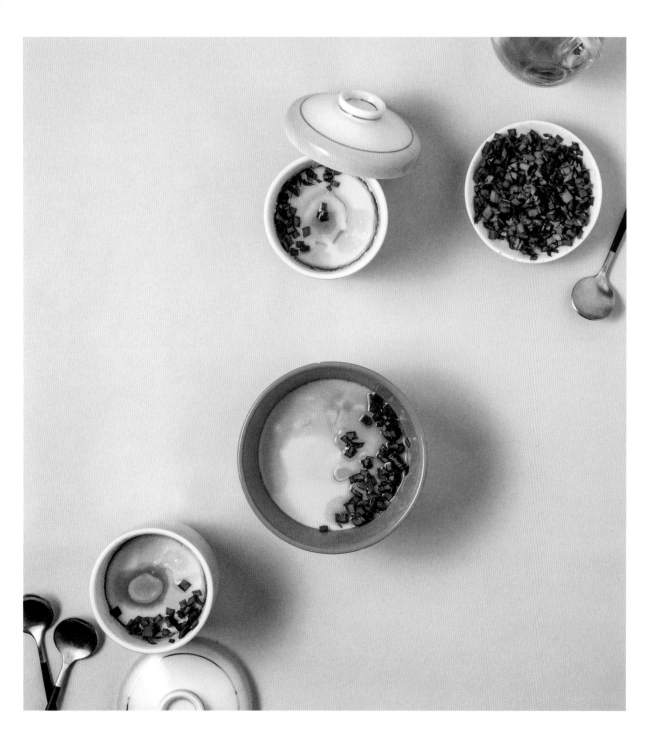

NUTRITION FACTS: **Full Recipe:** 385 calories, 28 g fat, 2.7 g total carbs, 0.1 g fiber (2.62 g net carbs), 27.2 g protein
Per Serving: 192 calories, 14.2 g fat, 1.3 g total carbs, 0 g fiber (1.3 g total carbs), 13.6 g protein

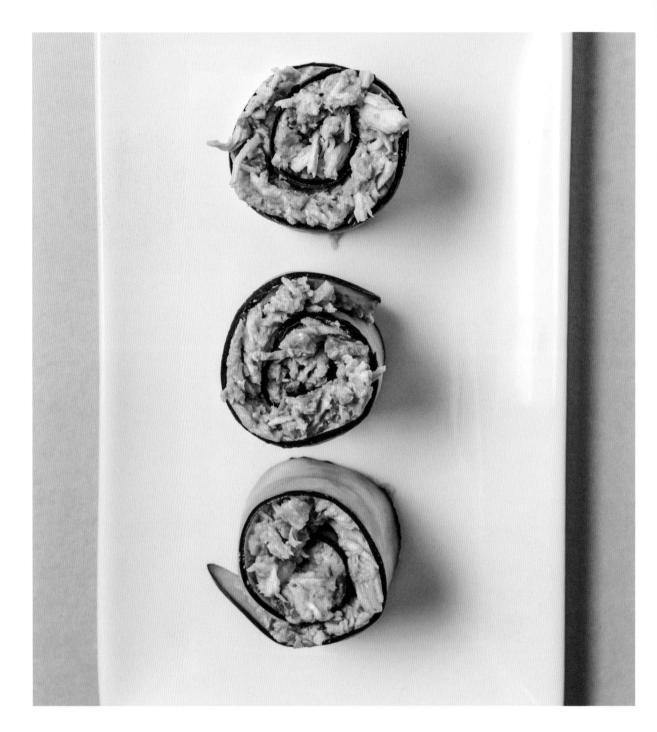

NUTRITION FACTS: **Full Recipe:** 845 calories, 55 g fat, 29.1 g total carbs,
11.9 g fiber (17.24 g net carbs), 66.1 g protein
Per Serving: 211 calories, 13.7 g fat, 7.3 g total carbs,
3 g fiber (4.31 g net carbs), 16.5 g protein

Chicken Salad Cucumber Roll-Up

YIELD: 4 servings (16 rolls)
SERVING SIZE: 4 rolls

PREP TIME: 15 minutes
TOTAL TIME: 15 minutes

With precooked ingredients, this recipe is as simple as mixing and rolling! Cucumber roll-ups make a great lunch or snack, and they are incredibly versatile. You can stuff them with a variety of different ingredients—tuna, salmon, turkey, or the like—tailored to suit your tastes, or use whatever you have on hand.

INGREDIENTS:

2 large cucumbers, thinly sliced lengthwise

8 ounces (225 g) cooked rotisserie chicken meat, chopped or shredded

2 slices cooked bacon, crumbled (or use 2 tablespoons [14 g] prepackaged bacon crumbles)

½ avocado, mashed

1 tablespoon (14 g) mayonnaise (see page 249)

1 teaspoon sesame seeds

1 teaspoon lime juice (optional)

salt to taste

INSTRUCTIONS:

1. Lay cucumber slices out flat across paper towels to absorb excess moisture.

2. Combine chicken, bacon, avocado, mayonnaise, sesame seeds, and lime juice, if using. Taste mixture and season with salt to taste.

3. Spread a small amount of chicken mixture onto a cucumber slice. Roll the cucumber into a spiral shape to encase the mixture.

4. Repeat with remaining cucumber slices. Serve immediately.

NOTE: Lime juice will help prevent the avocado from browning, but it is optional if you intend to eat right away!

Calamari "Udon" Noodle Soup

YIELD: 2 servings
SERVING SIZE: 2½ cups (570 ml)

PREP TIME: 10 minutes
COOK TIME: 45 minutes

TOTAL TIME: 55 minutes

Although some seafood has a higher carbohydrate content than other meats, such as beef, pork, or poultry, it can still be enjoyed on a keto diet. Squid, or calamari, is a perfect example of this! In 100 grams of squid, there are 1.87 g of carbs—this is still firmly planted in the realm of keto-compatible foods. Don't fret the carbs when eating seafood, but be mindful of how they can add up when consumed in large amounts.

If you're searching for something a little more adventurous than your standard veggie noodle, this recipe is for you! Cut into thin ribbons and slowly cooked in a rich broth, the squid takes on a texture similar to udon noodles. Squid is one of my all-time favorite noodle substitutes, and it's jam-packed with protein.

INGREDIENTS:

3 stalks green onion

2 cups (475 ml) beef broth

2 cups (475 ml) water

1 teaspoon coconut aminos or soy sauce

8 ounces (225 g) squid tubes or rings, fresh or frozen, thawed

½ teaspoon fish sauce

2 soft-boiled eggs

½ cup (32 g) enoki mushrooms (or mushroom of choice)

4 sprigs fresh Thai basil

¼ teaspoon sesame seeds

INSTRUCTIONS:

1. Cut 1 stalk of green onion into thin slivers and reserve for garnish.

2. Combine remaining green onion, beef broth, 2 cups (475 ml) ofwater, and coconut aminos in a large stockpot. Bring to a boil and then reduce heat to low.

3. Clean squid tubes and remove membrane if necessary. Cut along one side of each tube to lay squid flat. Using a sharp knife, cut squid lengthwise into ¼ inch (6 mm)–thick ribbons or noodle shapes. Add squid to pot, gently stir to separate squid noodles, cover, and cook for 45 minutes.

4. Remove pot from heat, discard green onion, and stir fish sauce into broth.

5. Divide soup and squid noodles evenly between two serving bowls. Divide soft-boiled eggs, mushrooms, and Thai basil into bowls. Garnish with sesame seeds and green onion. Serve immediately.

NOTE: When cooked properly, squid is incredibly tender. It requires either a quick cook at high temperature or a slow cook over low heat—the areas in between can result in an undesirable chewy texture.

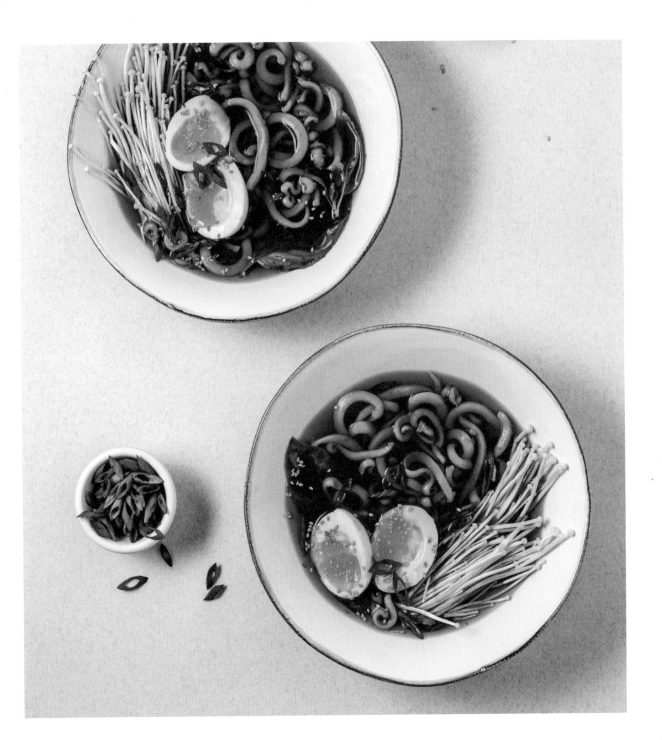

NUTRITION FACTS: **Full Recipe:** 422 calories, 14 g fat, 16.4 g total carbs, 1.6 g fiber (14.8 g net carbs), 53 g protein
Per Serving: 210 calories, 7 g fat, 8.2 g total carbs, 0.8 g fiber (7.4 g net carbs), 26.6 g protein

Italian Egg Drop Soup

YIELD: 4 servings (8 cups [1.9 L])
SERVING SIZE: 2 cups (475 ml)

PREP TIME: 3 minutes
COOK TIME: 20 minutes

TOTAL TIME: 23 minutes

I'm *obsessed* with this soup. Thin rags of egg and spinach in a savory broth make for a surprisingly satiating meal that's low in carbs and calories. Serve it as a side dish or the main course on chilly days when nothing sounds better than warm, nourishing soup.

INGREDIENTS:

1 teaspoon avocado oil or cooking fat of choice

½ medium onion, diced

8 cups (1.9 L) chicken broth

6 eggs

2 tablespoons (18 g) nutritional yeast

¼ teaspoon salt

¼ teaspoon dried parsley

2 cups (60 g) baby spinach leaves

INSTRUCTIONS:

1. In a large stock pot, heat avocado oil over medium high heat. Add onion and cook until translucent. Add chicken broth, stir, and bring to a boil. Reduce heat to low medium and cook broth for 10 to 15 minutes.

2. While broth is cooking, whisk eggs, nutritional yeast, salt, and parsley in a large pourable measuring cup or container with spout until completely smooth. Inspect for large lumps and break up with a utensil if needed.

3. Stir broth in one circular direction while slowly drizzling in egg mixture to form thin shreds of egg.

4. Remove from heat and mix in spinach. Salt to taste and serve immediately.

NOTE: If you have fresh parsley on hand, feel free to substitute it for the dried ingredient and use it for garnish.

If dairy is well tolerated, grated Parmesan cheese can substitute for nutritional yeast if you prefer.

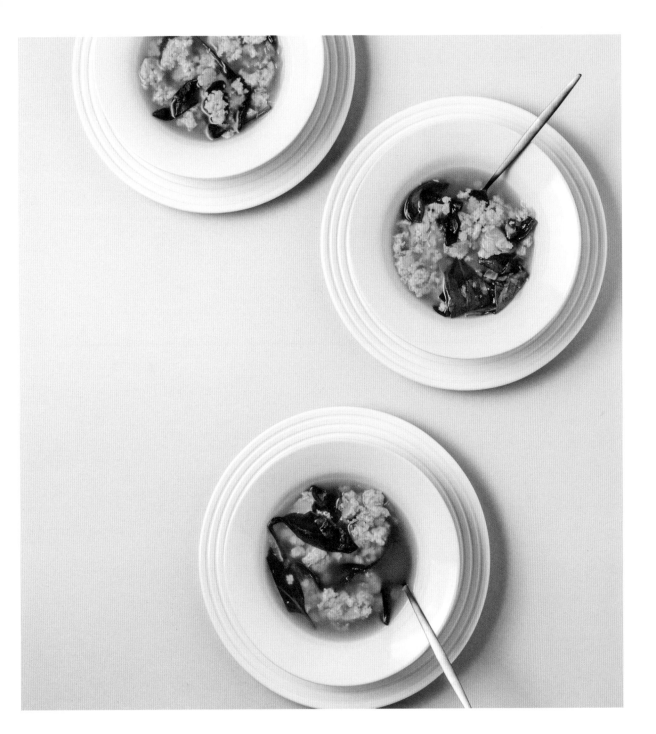

NUTRITION FACTS: **Full Recipe:** 685 calories, 36 g fat, 22.5 g total carbs,
6.2 g fiber (16.38 g net carbs), 64 g protein
Per Serving: 171 calories, 9 g fat, 5.6 total carbs,
1.5 g fiber (4.10 g net carbs), 16 g protein

Coconut Curry Stew

YIELD: 4 servings
SERVING SIZE: about 2½ cups (570 ml, or ¼ of the recipe)

PREP TIME: 10 minutes
COOK TIME: 30 minutes
TOTAL TIME: 40 minutes

Soups and stews are simple meals to make, and they offer an easy way to load up on nutrient-dense ingredients. This hearty coconut curry stew, perfect for a cold day, is loaded with nourishing micronutrients! It's low in carbs and rich in vitamin A, B vitamins, vitamin C, potassium, calcium, and magnesium.

INGREDIENTS:

1 teaspoon ghee or cooking fat of choice

¼ medium onion, diced

1 pound (455 g) boneless, skinless chicken breast, thinly sliced and cut to 1-inch (2.5 cm) length

2 medium turnips, cubed

4 ounces (115 g) collard greens, tough stems removed

2 tablespoons (30 g) red curry paste

1 teaspoon fresh, grated ginger

4 cups (946 ml) chicken broth

1 can (13.6 ounces, or 382 ml) of coconut milk

1 stalk lemon grass, smashed

salt to taste

INSTRUCTIONS:

1. In a large stock pot, cook fat and onion over medium high heat. When onions become translucent, add chicken, turnip, collard greens, red curry paste, and ginger. Cook for 2 to 3 minutes.

2. Stir in chicken broth, coconut milk, and smashed lemongrass stalk to stock pot. Bring to a boil. Bring down to a gentle simmer by reducing to low heat, cover with lid, and cook for an additional 20 to 30 minutes.

3. Remove from heat, carefully remove lemongrass stalk, and salt to taste. Serve.

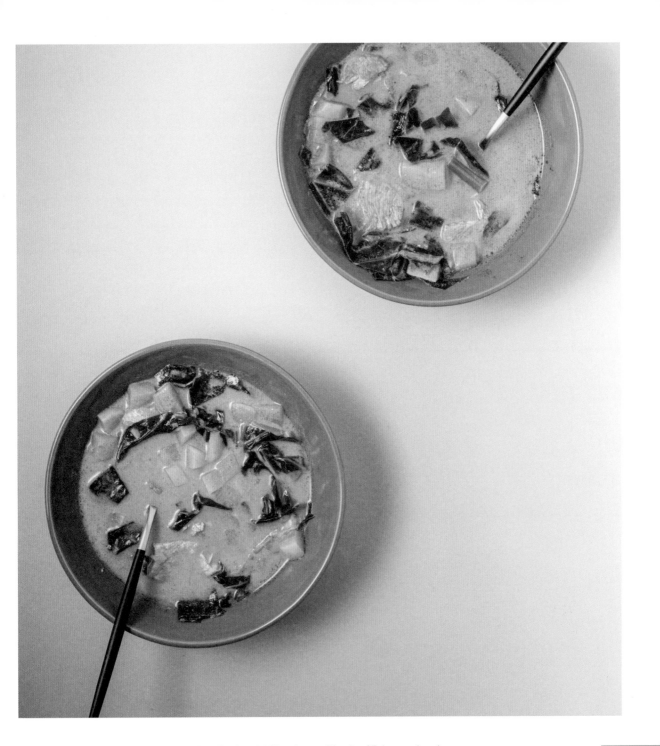

NUTRITION FACTS: **Full Recipe:** 1,643 calories, 89 g fat, 37.6 g total carbs, 10.6 g fiber (27.1 g net carbs), 158.2 g protein
Per Serving: 411 calories, 22.2 g fat, 9.4 g total carbs, 2.6 g fiber (6.76 g net carbs), 39.6 g protein

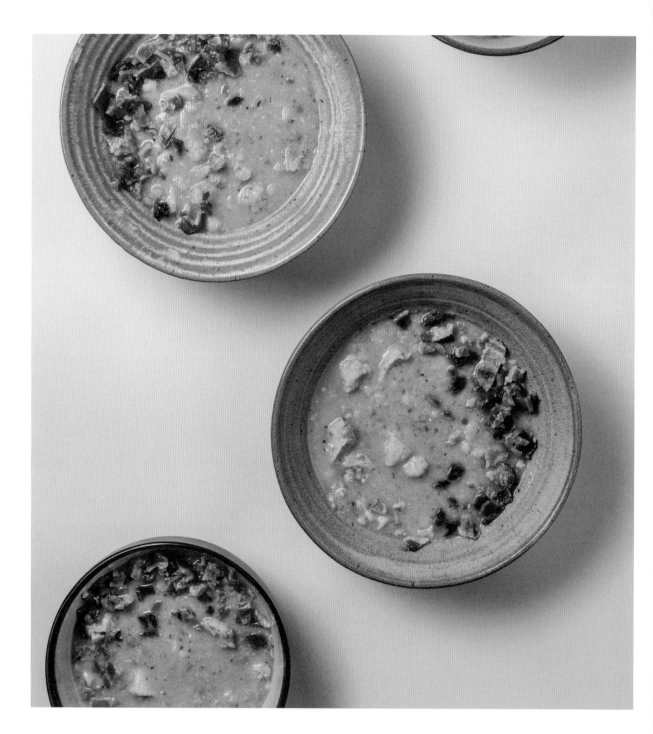

NUTRITION FACTS: **Full Recipe:** 1,806 calories, 93.2 g fat, 36.4 g total carbs, 12.6 g fiber (23.79 g net carbs), 198.5 g protein
Per Serving: 301 calories, 15.5 g fat, 6.1 g total carbs, 2.1 g fiber (3.96 g net carbs), 33.1 g protein

Hearty Chicken Chowder

YIELD: 6 servings
SERVING SIZE: 1½ cups (355 ml)

PREP TIME: 10 minutes
COOK TIME: 20 minutes

TOTAL TIME: 30 minutes

This chowder is so thick and creamy, you would never guess that it is completely dairy-free! The base of the recipe is incredibly versatile, making it easy to swap in different proteins and flavor profiles or add in more vegetables.

INGREDIENTS:

4 cups (946 ml) chicken stock

1 head medium cauliflower, cut into florets

½ pound (225 g) bacon, minced

¼ medium onion

1 pound (455 g) chicken breast, cut into ½-inch (2.5 cm) cubes

1 teaspoon dried oregano

1 teaspoon red chili flakes

salt to taste

ground black pepper to taste

INSTRUCTIONS:

1. Place chicken stock and half of cauliflower florets in a large stock pot. Bring to a boil and then reduce to a simmer over medium-low heat.

2. In a large skillet, cook bacon and onion over medium heat until fat renders. Add chicken breast, oregano, red chili flakes, and remaining cauliflower florets to the pan. Cook until chicken is no longer pink in the center and cauliflower is tender.

3. Remove chicken stock mixture from heat. Using a handheld immersion blender, puree the mixture. Once thoroughly blended, stir in the contents of the skillet.

4. Return to heat source and simmer for an additional 5 minutes. Season with salt and pepper to taste. Remove from heat and serve.

NOTE: If you prefer dairy-based chowder and tolerate it well, you can add half-and-half (lower calories) or heavy cream (higher fat and calories) to the chicken stock and cauliflower mixture prior to blending. Alternatively, you can mix shredded cheese into the chowder when adding the contents of the skillet.

No-Bean Chili

YIELD: 6 servings (approx. 8 cups [1.9 L])
SERVING SIZE: 1⅓ cups (315 ml, or ⅙ of the recipe)

PREP TIME: 10 minutes
COOK TIME: 4 hours
TOTAL TIME: 4 hours 10 minutes

Simple and delicious, this keto-friendly cowboy chili lightens the carb load by leaving out the beans. Let it cook slowly on the stovetop or in a slow cooker for a big family dinner or meal prep. It's even better as leftovers!

INGREDIENTS:

2 strips bacon, minced

½ medium onion, diced

4 cloves garlic, minced

2 pounds (900 g) top round beef, cut into 1-inch (2.5 cm) cubes

1 cup (235 ml) brewed coffee

1 cup (235 ml) beef broth

4 tablespoons (30 g) chili powder

1 tablespoon (7 g) cumin

1 tablespoon (7 g) smoked paprika

1 teaspoon salt to taste

½ teaspoon ground black pepper

INSTRUCTIONS:

1. In a large enameled Dutch oven or stock pot with fitted lid, cook bacon over medium heat until fat begins to render. Add onion and cook until translucent. Add garlic and beef, mixing until the meat has browned evenly.

2. Pour coffee and beef broth into the pan. Using a wooden spoon, scrape any residual onion, garlic, or meat from the bottom of the pan.

3. Stir in chili powder, cumin, smoked paprika, salt, and pepper. Increase heat to high and bring to a boil. Once the mixture is boiling, drop heat to medium-low and cover.

4. Remove lid to stir periodically and assess fluid level as the chili reduces. If fluid is evaporating too quickly, reduce heat to low and cover. Add water as needed to reach desired consistency.

5. After 4 hours, give chili a final stir, breaking up the tender chunks of meat into smaller bits. Salt to taste and serve.

NOTE: This recipe can also be prepared in a slow cooker set to low for 8 to 10 hours, or high for 4 to 6 hours.

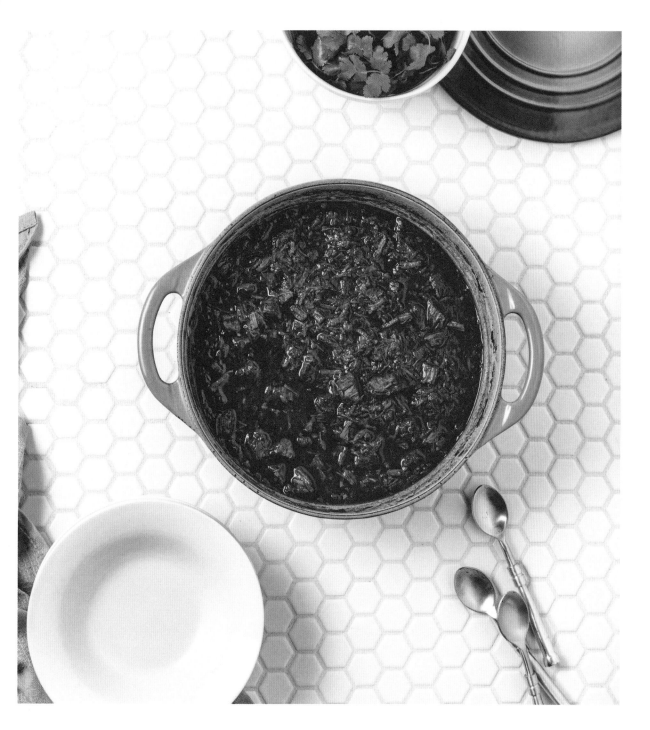

NUTRITION FACTS: **Full Recipe:** 1,699 calories, 52.5 g fat, 30.8 g total carbs, 14.2 g fiber (16.56 g net carbs), 285.8 g protein
Per Serving: 283 calories, 8.7 g fat, 5.1 g total carbs, 2.4 g fiber (2.76 g net carbs), 47.64 g protein

Keto "Macaroni and Cheese"

YIELD: 6 servings
SERVING SIZE: approx. 1½ cups
  (300 g, or ⅙ of the recipe)

SOAKING TIME: 8 hours
PREP TIME: 10 minutes
COOK TIME: 20 minutes

TOTAL TIME: 8 hours 30 minutes

Without macaroni noodles or cheese, calling this recipe "macaroni and cheese" is undoubtedly a bit of a stretch. I'm not so bold to suggest that this will fool your taste buds into believing it is the real deal. However, this recipe is a great example of how old favorites can inspire lower carb versions and how ingredients you may be trying to avoid can ultimately be replaced with more healthful options. Although this is neither macaroni, nor cheese, the result is quite delicious.

SPECIAL DIET CONSIDERATIONS: Contains nuts.

INGREDIENTS:

½ cup (70 g) cashews

¼ cup (8 g) nutritional yeast

1 teaspoon garlic powder

½ teaspoon mustard powder

1½ cups (355 ml) unflavored, unsweetened almond, macadamia, or hemp seed, or other nut milk of choice

1 medium head cauliflower, chopped

1 pound (455 g) uncured ham, chopped

salt to taste

INSTRUCTIONS:

1. Soak cashews in water overnight. Discard water.

2. Place soaked cashews in food processor with nutritional yeast, garlic powder, mustard powder, and milk. Blend.

3. Preheat oven to 400°F (200°C or gas mark 6).

4. Arrange cauliflower and ham on a large baking sheet. Bake for 10 to 15 minutes.

5. Heat cashew mixture in a large saucepan or stockpot over low heat to thicken, whisking occasionally.

6. Stir baked cauliflower and ham into the cashew mixture. Salt to taste and serve.

NOTE: This recipe describes how to make a dairy-free "cheese" sauce; however, if dairy is well tolerated, you can use a more traditional cheese sauce recipe if you prefer!

NUTRITION FACTS:

Full Recipe: 1,139 calories, 54.5 g fat, 69.4 g total carbs, 18.3 g fiber (51.10 g net carbs), 118.9 g protein
Per Serving: 190 calories, 9.1 g fat, 11.6 g total carbs, 3 g fiber (8.52 g net carbs), 19.8 g protein

Baked Chicken Tenders with Fries

YIELD: 6 servings
SERVING SIZE: ⅙ of the recipe

PREP TIME: 15 minutes
COOK TIME: 60 minutes

TOTAL TIME: 1 hour 15 minutes

Low-carb breading and jicama in place of potatoes makes this traditional comfort food low in carbohydrates and suitable for a standard ketogenic diet.

INGREDIENTS:

Fries

1 medium jicama

1 tablespoon (15 ml) olive oil or cooking oil of your choice

salt to taste

Chicken Tenders

2 tablespoons (24 g) psyllium husk powder

¼ cup (28 g) flaxseed meal

1 teaspoon paprika

1 teaspoon dried oregano

⅛ teaspoon salt

1½ pounds (680 g) boneless, skinless chicken tenderloins, or breast meat cut into strips

1 tablespoon (15 g) mayonnaise (see page 249)

INSTRUCTIONS:

1. Preheat oven to 400°F (200°C or gas mark 6).

2. Clean and peel jicama. Carefully slice jicama into ¼-inch (6 mm) disks. Cut these disks lengthwise into ¼ inch (6 mm)–thick strips to make the fries.

3. Transfer jicama fries to a large baking sheet. Evenly coat the fries by tossing them in olive oil and season with salt. Place baking sheet in oven and bake for approximately 50 to 60 minutes, depending on desired crispness.

4. While the fries bake, combine psyllium husk powder, flaxseed meal, paprika, oregano, and salt in a large dish.

5. Place a baking rack on a baking tray.

6. Cover chicken in mayonnaise and then dredge each piece of chicken in the flaxseed meal mixture. Using tongs, carefully transfer each piece of chicken to the prepared baking tray.

7. With 15 to 20 minutes left to bake on jicama fries, carefully place baking tray with chicken into the oven. Bake 15 to 20 minutes or until chicken has fully cooked. Remove both trays from the oven and serve.

NOTE: As an alternative to psyllium husk powder and flaxseed meal, you can use crushed pork rinds in their place to further reduce the total carbohydrate count if needed. Pork rinds also add a nice crunch similar to crispy fried chicken!

NUTRITION FACTS:

Full Recipe: 2,210 calories, 112 g fat, 110.4 g total carbs, 65.5 g fiber (44.86 g net carbs), 187.4 g protein
Per Serving: 368 calories, 18.8 g fat, 18.4 g total carbs, 10.9 g fiber (7.48 g net carbs), 31.2 g protein

Chicken and Waffles

YIELD: 4 servings (8 small waffles)
SERVING SIZE: 2 waffles with ¼ of the gravy

PREP TIME: 5 minutes
COOK TIME: 15 minutes
TOTAL TIME: 20 minutes

A savory chicken and veggie gravy over low-carb waffles is a healthy departure from traditional chicken and waffles. If you're in the mood for something sweet, feel free to garnish the waffles with berries instead!

INGREDIENTS:

Waffles

2 large eggs, separated

¼ cup (60 ml) unsweetened coconut milk

dash salt

½ cup (56 g) finely ground almond flour

¼ teaspoon baking powder

8 sprays coconut oil nonstick spray or nonstick spray of your choice

Chicken Gravy

1 tablespoon (14 g) ghee or cooking fat of your choice

8 ounces (225 g) chicken breast, cubed

½ cup (50 g) cut green beans

½ medium red bell pepper, diced

2 tablespoons (28 ml) coconut milk

salt to taste

INSTRUCTIONS:

1. Preheat waffle iron.

2. In a large mixing bowl, combine egg yolks and coconut milk until mixture is smooth.

3. In a small mixing bowl, combine salt, almond flour, and baking powder. Whisk dry ingredients into the egg mixture until smooth.

4. In a separate bowl, beat the egg whites with an electric hand mixer until soft peaks form. Gently fold egg whites into the batter.

5. Spray coconut oil on the surface of the hot waffle iron prior to adding batter. Pour batter (approximately 2 tablespoons [28 ml] of batter for each waffle) onto waffle iron and close. Cook each waffle about 2 to 3 minutes until golden brown. Carefully remove and keep warm.

6. Melt ghee in skillet over medium high heat. Add chicken breast and cook until no longer pink in the center.

7. Scrape down sides of pan with spatula and mix in green beans, red bell pepper, and coconut milk. Cook for 2 to 3 minutes to reduce moisture and thicken gravy. Season with salt and remove from heat.

8. Serve waffles with chicken gravy over the top.

NOTE: The amount of batter required per waffle may vary based on the size and model of the waffle iron.

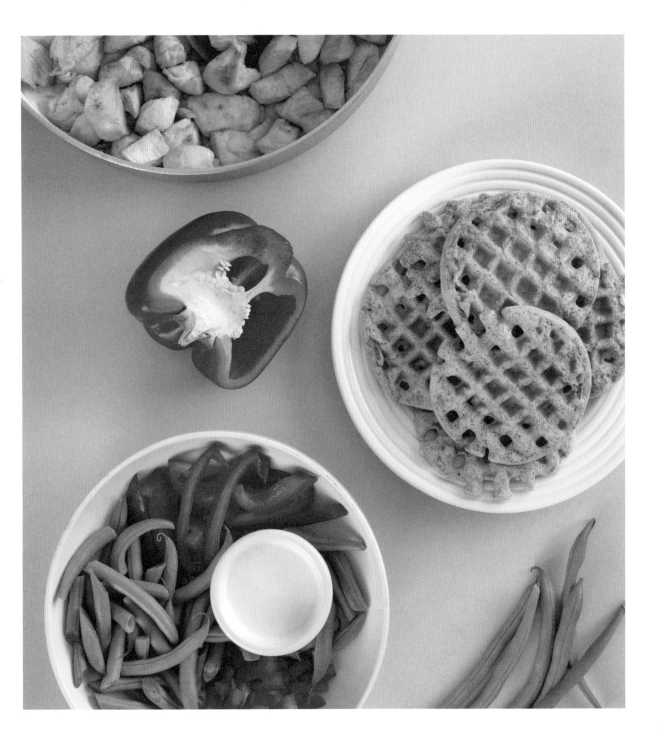

NUTRITION FACTS:　　**Full Recipe:** 1,009 calories, 69.6 g fat, 20.5 g total carbs,
8.6 g fiber (11.93 g net carbs), 77.2 g protein
Per Serving: 252 calories, 17.4 g fat, 5.1 g total carbs,
2.2 g fiber (2.98 g net carbs), 19.3 g protein

—
215

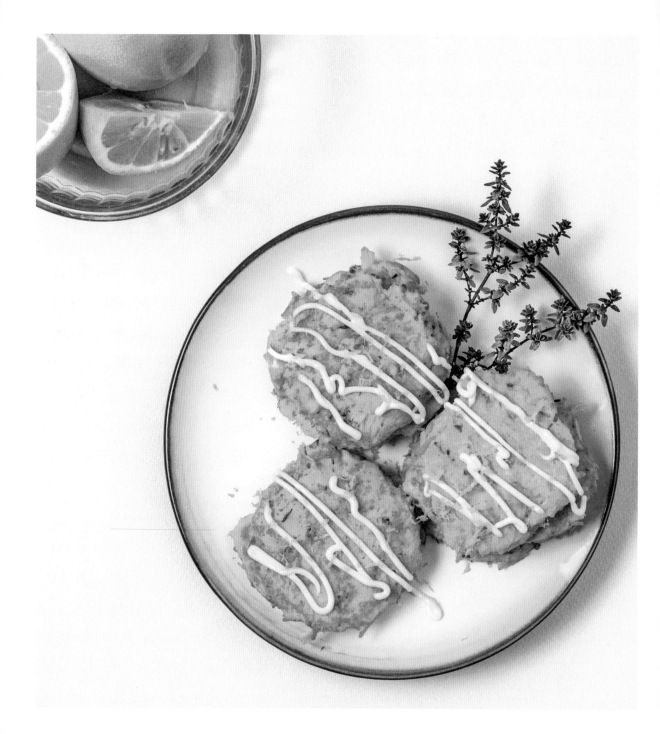

NUTRITION FACTS: **Full Recipe:** 750 calories, 47 g fat, 4.5 g total carbs, 1.2 g fiber (3.33 g net carbs), 74 g protein
Per Serving: 375 calories, 23.4 g fat, 2.3 g total carbs, 0.6 g fiber (1.67 g net carbs), 37 g protein

Mustard Thyme Chicken Fritters

YIELD: 2 servings
SERVING SIZE: 5 fritters (half of the recipe)

PREP TIME: 5 minutes
COOK TIME: 10 minutes
TOTAL TIME: 15 minutes

Fritters are one of my absolute favorite things to whip up when I'm feeling like a hot meal but don't have much time to cook. You can use any kind of precooked meat, seafood, or even grated veggies with different herbs and spices to add variety.

INGREDIENTS:

8 ounces (225 g) cooked, shredded chicken breast

2 tablespoons (30 g) mayonnaise (see page 249)

2 tablespoons (30 g) Dijon mustard

1 teaspoon dried thyme

salt to taste

1 egg

Sauce

1 tablespoon (15 g) mayonnaise

1 teaspoon lemon juice

INSTRUCTIONS:

1. Heat a skillet or griddle to medium-low heat.

2. Combine chicken, mayonnaise, mustard, and thyme in a small bowl. Taste mixture and season with salt to taste.

3. Beat in egg until the mixture is smooth and evenly blended.

4. Using a spoon, transfer 1-ounce (28 g) portions of mixture to the hot pan, giving enough space to each portion to easily flip. Press mixture into a flat circle and cook for 2 to 3 minutes or until lightly browned. Gently flip each fritter and cook for an additional 2 minutes on the other side. Place on a warm plate to rest.

5. While fritters are cooking, whisk together mayonnaise and lemon juice.

6. Drizzle lemon mayo over top of finished fritters and serve immediately.

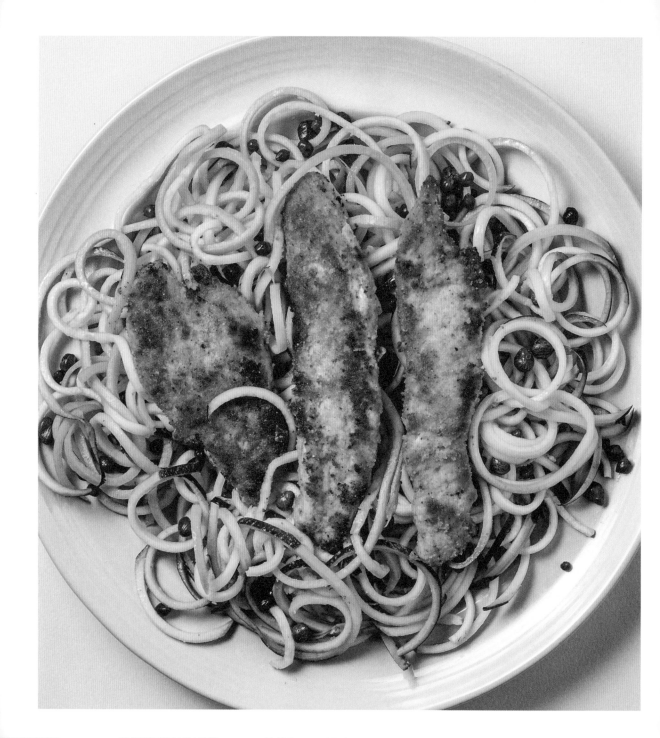

NUTRITION FACTS: **Full Recipe:** 1,963 calories, 84 g fat, 35.1 g total carbs,
11.6 g fiber (23.46 g net carbs), 263.7 g protein
Per Serving: 327 calories, 14 g fat, 5.9 g total carbs,
1.9 g fiber (3.91 g net carbs), 43.9 g protein

Chicken Piccata with Squash Noodles

YIELD: 6 servings
SERVING SIZE: ⅙ of the recipe

PREP TIME: 10 minutes
COOK TIME: 20 minutes

TOTAL TIME: 30 minutes

Almond flour and veggie noodles give this classic dish a low carb twist.

SPECIAL DIET CONSIDERATIONS: Ghee is clarified butter, which means it contains dairy. Though the milk proteins will largely be removed, if you have a dairy sensitivity or allergy, you may want to use an alternative cooking fat to replace the ghee in this recipe.

INGREDIENTS:

2 medium to large summer squash or zucchini

4 boneless, skinless chicken breast halves

½ cup (56 g) almond flour or meal

½ teaspoon salt

¼ teaspoon ground black pepper

2 tablespoons (28 g) ghee or cooking fat of choice

½ cup (120 ml) chicken broth

3 tablespoons (45 ml) lemon juice

¼ cup (34 g) capers

INSTRUCTIONS:

1. Cut summer squash into long noodle-like strands using a spiralizer tool or julienne peeler. Place squash noodles on large plate lined with paper towels to absorb excess moisture until ready to cook.

2. Butterfly chicken breast halves. Using a meat tenderizer, pound the chicken into approximately ¼ inch (6 mm)–thick pieces.

3. Combine almond flour, salt, and pepper on a dish. Dredge each piece of chicken in flour mixture to coat.

4. Heat ghee over medium high heat in a large skillet and add dredged chicken pieces. Cook until each side has browned, approximately 3 minutes on each side, and chicken is cooked through. Remove chicken from skillet and keep warm.

5. To the pan, add chicken broth, lemon juice, and capers. Scrape browned chicken pieces and remaining breading from the sides of the pan with a spatula and mix ingredients together. Bring the sauce to a boil and allow the sauce to reduce to thicken. Turn heat to low.

6. Toss squash noodles in sauce over low heat for 1 to 2 minutes. Remove from heat and plate with cooked chicken. Serve immediately.

NOTE: If summer squash is out of season or otherwise unavailable, try substituting spaghetti squash for the vegetable noodles.

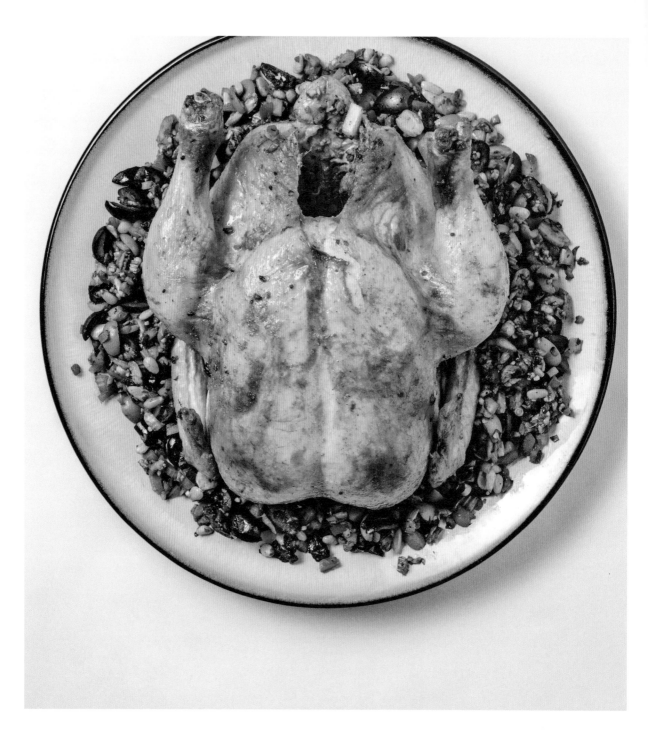

NUTRITION FACTS: **Full Recipe:** 3,618 calories, 267.7 g fat, 32.8 g total carbs, 12.8 g fiber (20 g net carbs), 259.4 g protein
Per Serving: 603 calories, 44.6 g fat, 5.5 g total carbs, 2.1 g fiber (3.34 g net carbs), 43.2 g protein

Roasted Chicken with Celery Olive Stuffing

YIELD: 6 servings
SERVING SIZE: ⅙ of the recipe

PREP TIME: 15 minutes
COOK TIME: 1 hour 10 minutes

RESTING TIME: 20 minutes
TOTAL TIME: 1 hour 45 minutes

Although there is certainly nothing wrong with premade rotisserie chicken, roasting your own chicken is quite easy. The DIY route opens up creative flavor combinations and the payoff for the extra effort is spectacular! If you aren't feeding a large family for dinner, portion out the carved chicken for meal prep or use the leftovers for soups and casseroles.

SPECIAL DIET CONSIDERATIONS: Contains nuts. Omit pine nuts if allergic.

INGREDIENTS:

1 whole 3-pound (1.4 kg) chicken, skin on

½ teaspoon ground coriander

½ teaspoon ground cumin

½ teaspoon olive oil

¼ teaspoon salt

2 cloves garlic, minced

½ cup (70 g) quartered black olives

½ cup (70 g) quartered kalamata olives

½ cup (70 g) quartered green olives

4 stalks celery, chopped

4 large button mushrooms, diced

¼ cup (35 g) pine nuts

¼ lemon, cut in wedges

INSTRUCTIONS:

1. Preheat oven to 350°F (180°C or gas mark 4).

2. Remove giblets and neck from chicken; discard or save for another use. Pat chicken dry using paper towels. Slide fingers under the chicken skin at the openings to loosen skin and create deep pockets for seasoning.

3. Combine coriander, cumin, olive oil, salt, and half of the garlic. Spread paste over the chicken meat underneath the skin. Season outside of skin with any remaining spice mixture.

4. Combine remaining garlic with olives, celery, mushrooms, and pine nuts. Stuff the mixture inside the cavity of the chicken along with lemon wedges. Optional: truss the chicken with cooking twine, securing the legs and wings close to the body for a more even cook.

5. Place chicken on a roasting pan, breast-side up.

6. Bake for 1 hour 10 minutes or until internal temperature of chicken and stuffing has reached a minimum of 180°F (82°C). Baste chicken every 20 minutes with the drippings.

7. Remove from heat, cover with aluminum foil, and let rest for 20 to 30 minutes prior to serving.

8. Remove stuffing from the cavity and serve alongside carved chicken.

Pan-Seared Duck

YIELD: 4 servings
SERVING SIZE: ¼ of the recipe

PREP TIME: 10 minutes
COOK TIME: 30 minutes

TOTAL TIME: 40 minutes

Don't be intimidated by cooking duck breast—it's incredibly simple and packed full of flavor!

INGREDIENTS:

1 pound (455 g) duck breast halves

sea salt to taste

ground black pepper to taste

1 clove garlic, minced

2 tablespoons (20 g) minced shallots

1 tablespoon (7 g) coconut flour

1 tablespoon (15 ml) apple cider vinegar

1 cup (235 ml) chicken broth

2 tablespoons (5 g) minced fresh basil

2 daikon radishes, spiralized or julienned

1 cup (30 g) baby spinach

INSTRUCTIONS:

1. Preheat oven to 425°F (220°C or gas mark 7) and heat a large oven-safe skillet over medium heat.

2. Using a sharp knife, carefully score a crosshatch pattern into the skin and fat of the duck breast, taking care not to cut into the meat. Pat the duck breasts dry with paper towels. Season with salt and pepper.

3. Brown duck breasts skin-side down on the hot skillet and cook for 5 minutes to render fat. Flip each breast and sear for 1 minute. Carefully draw off duck fat and reserve and then place pan in the oven and bake for 10 to 12 minutes or until the internal temperature reaches desired level of doneness. The USDA recommends a safe minimum temperature of 165°F (74°C).

4. Remove duck breast from oven and let rest on cutting board for 5 to 10 minutes. Thinly slice breasts approximately ¼-inch (6 mm) thick when ready to serve.

5. Return duck fat to skillet and heat over medium high heat. Add garlic and shallots; scrape down browned bits stuck to the pan and incorporate them into the mixture. Whisk in coconut flour until mixture is uniform in appearance. Slowly whisk in vinegar, then chicken broth. Continue whisking over heat until sauce thickens.

6. Once sauce thickens, stir in basil and reduce heat to low.

7. Toss daikon radishes and baby spinach in the sauce until spinach wilts and daikon softens, about two minutes. Salt to taste.

8. Serve daikon noodles and sauce alongside sliced duck breast.

NUTRITION FACTS:

Full Recipe: 1,104 calories, 47 g fat, 37.5 g total carbs, 14.8 g fiber (22.71 g net carbs), 127.4 g protein
Per Serving: 276 calories, 11.8 g fat, 9.4 g total carbs, 3.7 g fiber (5.68 g net carbs), 31.8 g protein

Lamb-Stuffed Cabbage Rolls with Avgolemono Sauce

YIELD: 5 servings (15 cabbage rolls)
SERVING SIZE: 3 cabbage rolls and ⅕ of the sauce

PREP TIME: 20 minutes
COOK TIME: 40 minutes
TOTAL TIME: 1 hour

This recipe can be prepared in an hour or less, but most of it is active time. Cabbage rolls are a bit labor intensive, but they're so worth it! This can be a fun cooking project to do with kids, and the possible combinations for filling and sauces are truly endless. Traditional recipes use rice and other higher carb ingredients in the filling, but here we've swapped the rice out for minced celery!

INGREDIENTS:

Cabbage Rolls

1 large head green cabbage (using 15 leaves)

6 medium stalks celery, minced

¼ medium onion, minced

1 pound (455 g) ground lamb

1 egg

¼ teaspoon smoked paprika

¼ teaspoon salt

1 tablespoon (4 g) fresh dill, chopped

Avgolemono Sauce

1½ cups (355 ml) chicken broth or broth of choice

2 eggs, separated

1 tablespoon (15 ml) water

¼ cup (60 ml) lemon juice (1 large lemon, juiced)

INSTRUCTIONS:

Cabbage Rolls

1. Prepare a large stockpot of simmering water. Cut a deep, cone-shaped incision around bottom stem of cabbage to remove core. Place cabbage incision-side up in the simmering water, taking care to submerge most of the vegetable. As the cabbage cooks, the leaves will easily separate. Carefully remove individual leaves with tongs and set aside on a plate.

2. Sauté celery and onions over medium heat until onions become translucent. Transfer to a large mixing bowl.

3. Add lamb, egg, paprika, salt, and dill to the mixing bowl. Knead ingredients with hands until thoroughly combined.

4. To construct cabbage rolls, lay a cooked cabbage leaf on a cutting board and cut out the hard vein. Place approximately 1½ ounces (43 g) of lamb mixture toward the bottom of the leaf. Roll the bottom portion of the leaf over the meat, fold in the sides, and continue rolling to encase the filling. Place cabbage roll on a large steamer basket or rack. Line additional cabbage rolls in the basket in a single layer, side by side.

(continued)

(continued)

5. Pour 1 inch (2.5 cm) of water into a steamer pot with fitted lid. Place steamer basket or rack in the steamer. Cover with lid and steam for 25 to 30 minutes or until lamb is fully cooked to 160°F (71°C).

6. Place cabbage rolls in serving dish.

Avgolemono Sauce

1. As cabbage rolls are steaming, bring broth to a boil in a separate pan and then reduce heat to low.

2. In a large mixing bowl, whisk egg whites until soft peaks form.

3. Whisking continuously, very slowly add egg yolks, 1 tablespoon (15 ml) of water, lemon juice, and hot broth to ensure the ingredients smoothly blend together.

4. Pour sauce over top of the cabbage rolls in the dish, garnish with fresh dill, and serve.

NOTE: Alternatively, rather than steaming, the cabbage rolls can be baked at 400°F (200°C or gas mark 6) for 20 to 30 minutes.

Lamb can be replaced with any ground meat but cooking time and temperature goal may require adjustment.

The cabbage rolls also pair well with yogurt or tomato-based sauces, such as the Sugar-Free Spaghetti Sauce on page 247. Adjust the recipe to suit your tastes or experiment with different combinations!

NUTRITION FACTS:

Cabbage Rolls
Full Recipe: 1,505 calories, 96 g fat, 40.7 g total carbs, 16.1 g fiber (25.64 g net carbs), 117 g protein
Per Serving: 299 calories, 19 g fat, 7.8 g total carbs, 3.1 g fiber (4.69 g net carbs), 23 g protein

Avgolemono Sauce
Full Recipe: 176 calories, 9.9 g fat, 5.5 g total carbs, 0.1 g fiber (5.4 g net carbs), 15.7 g protein
Per Serving: 35 calories, 2 g fat, 1.1 g total carbs, 0 g fiber (1.1 g net carbs), 3.1 g protein

Cabbage Rolls with Avgolemono Sauce
Full Recipe: 1,681 calories, 106 g fat, 46.2 g total carbs, 16.2 g fiber (30 g net carbs), 132.7 g protein
Per Serving: 334 calories, 21 g fat, 8.9 g total carbs, 3.1 g fiber (5.8 g net carbs), 26.1 g protein

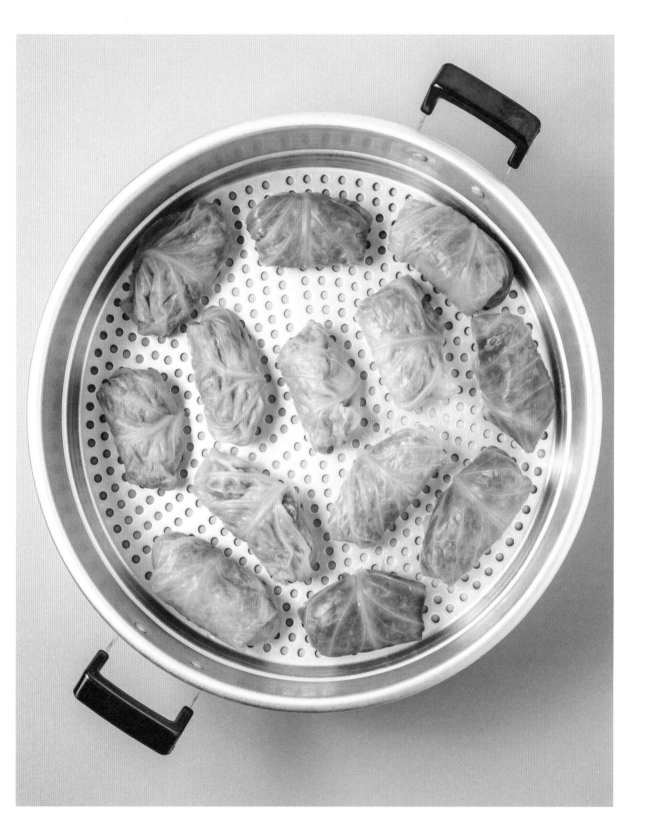

Roasted Red Cabbage and Pork Chops

YIELD: 6 servings
SERVING SIZE: ⅙ of the recipe

PREP TIME: 5 minutes
COOK TIME: 15 minutes

TOTAL TIME: 20 minutes

The sheet pan baking method makes quick work of this savory pork chop and cabbage dish. The combination of protein-rich pork with red cabbage and arugula delivers a lively flavor that is sure to please any palate!

INGREDIENTS:

1 tablespoon (15 ml) avocado oil or cooking fat of choice

1 tablespoon (15 ml) apple cider vinegar

½ medium head red cabbage, cut into 1-inch (2.5 cm) sections

3 ounces (85 g) prosciutto, thinly sliced

6 boneless loin pork chops (1 inch, or 2.5 cm thick)

¼ teaspoon garlic salt

⅛ teaspoon ground black pepper

1 cup (20 g) arugula

salt to taste

INSTRUCTIONS:

1. Preheat oven to 400°F (200°C or gas mark 6). Set a large sheet pan aside.

2. Place oil and vinegar into a large zipper lock bag. Place cabbage inside bag, zip, and lie flat to marinate for at least 5 minutes.

3. Line sheet pan with prosciutto. Place pork chops on top. Remove cabbage from marinade and distribute around and in between pork chops. Season pork with garlic salt and black pepper.

4. Place sheet pan in oven and bake for 10 minutes. Turn broiler to high and broil for 5 minutes to finish pork. Remove from oven and take internal temperature of pork to ensure it is fully cooked to a minimum of 145°F (63°C).

5. Garnish with arugula and salt to taste.

NOTE: Bone-in pork chops and thicker cuts of meat will require a slightly longer cook time. Increase time to ensure pork reaches an internal temperature of 145°F (63°C).

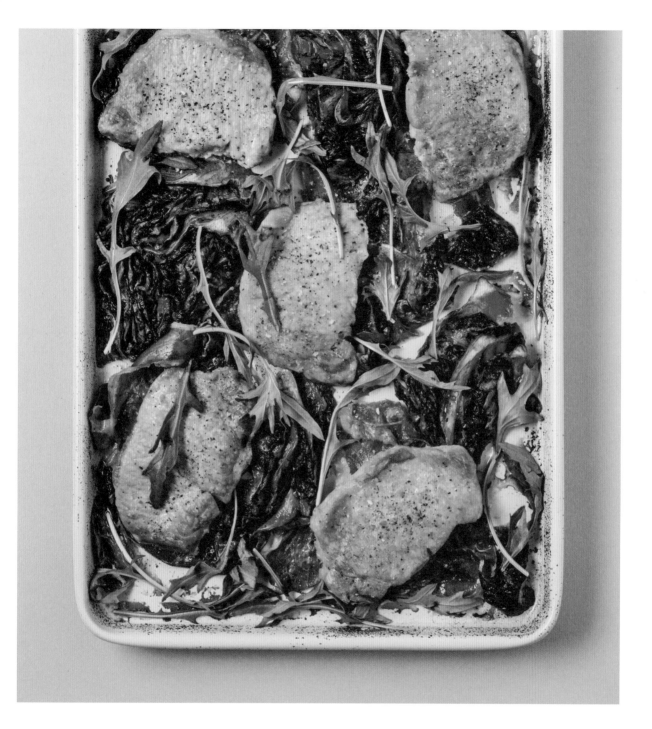

NUTRITION FACTS: **Full Recipe:** 1,422 calories, 70 g fat, 31.8 g total carbs,
9.2 g fiber (22.63 g net carbs), 162 g protein
Per Serving: 237 calories, 11.7 g fat, 5.3 g total carbs,
1.5 g fiber (3.77 g net carbs), 27 g protein

—

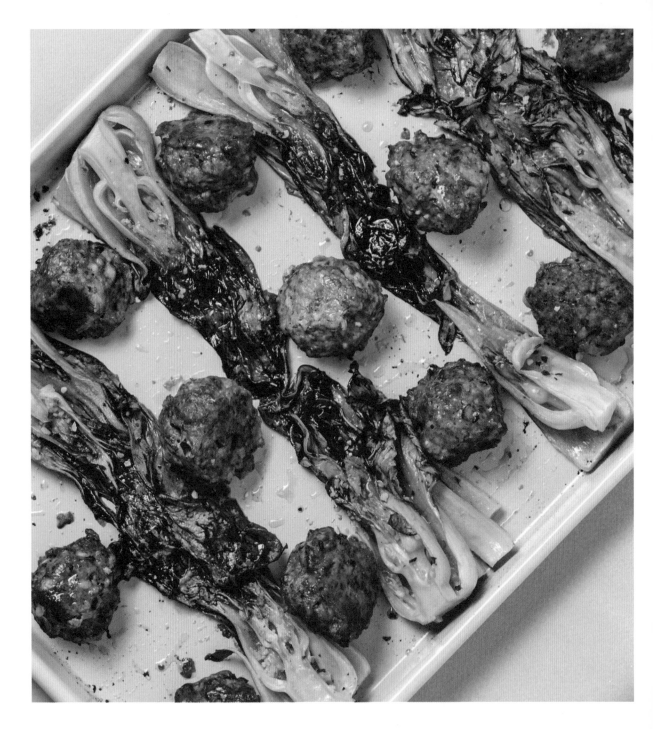

NUTRITION FACTS: **Full Recipe:** 1,774 calories, 130 g fat, 19 g total carbs, 5.3 g fiber (13.67 g net carbs), 136 g protein
Per Serving: 443 calories, 33 g fat, 4.7 g total carbs, 1.3 g fiber (3.42 g net carbs), 34 g protein

Sheet Pan Wonton Meatballs and Bok Choy

YIELD: 4 servings (16 meatballs)
SERVING SIZE: 4 meatballs and
 1 head bok choy

PREP TIME: 15 minutes
COOK TIME: 16 minutes
TOTAL TIME: 31 minutes

Here, mushroom and coconut flour replace the breadcrumbs and wheat flour found in traditional meatballs to reduce the carbs and increase the nutrient density. With each meatball bursting with umami flavor, this meal is a tried and true family favorite—even my kids love it!

INGREDIENTS:

Meatballs

1 pound (455 g) ground pork

1 teaspoon (8 g) fresh ginger, finely grated

2 large shiitake mushroom caps, minced

4 stalks green onion, minced

1 teaspoon coconut aminos or soy sauce

1 egg

½ tablespoon coconut flour

Bok Choy

4 heads baby bok choy

1 clove garlic, minced

2 tablespoons (28 ml) avocado oil

1 dash garlic salt

1 dash red pepper flakes

INSTRUCTIONS:

1. Preheat oven to 400°F (200°C or gas mark 6) and set aside a large sheet pan.

2. Combine pork, ginger, mushroom, onion, coconut aminos, and egg in a large bowl. Work coconut flour into the wet mixture until evenly distributed.

3. Form 1- to 1.5-ounce (28 to 43 g) meatballs with pork mixture and place on sheet pan spaced 2 inches (5 cm) apart.

4. Slice bok choy in half lengthwise and cut off the bottom portion. Thoroughly clean with running water and pat dry.

5. Combine garlic and avocado oil. Generously rub it over bok choy and into the leaves. Arrange bok choy around and between meatballs on the sheet pan. Sprinkle garlic salt and red pepper flakes over the vegetables.

6. Place sheet pan in oven to cook for 10 minutes. Carefully remove the sheet pan from the oven and flip each meatball using tongs. Place the sheet pan back into the oven for an additional 6 to 8 minutes or until meatballs are thoroughly cooked. Serve.

NOTE: Leftover meatballs can be frozen for reheating or made ahead and frozen for quick and easy meals.

Pork Tenderloin and Turnip Mash

YIELD: 4 servings
SERVING SIZE: ¼ of the recipe

PREP TIME: 30 minutes
COOK TIME: 45 minutes

TOTAL TIME: 1 hour 15 minutes

Cauliflower is a popular potato substitute for the standard keto diet, but there are plenty of other low carb vegetables that make suitable alternatives—radish, jicama, celeriac, and turnip, just to name a few! We'll use turnip to make creamy, sage-infused mashed "potatoes" in this recipe, paired with a savory pork tenderloin.

INGREDIENTS:

1½ pounds (680 g) pork tenderloin, visible fat and fascia trimmed

1 teaspoon yellow mustard

1 teaspoon garlic powder

1 teaspoon salt

1 teaspoon ground black pepper

1 pound (455 g) turnips, peeled and quartered

2 tablespoons (28 ml) olive oil

2 tablespoons (3 g) chopped fresh sage

salt to taste

INSTRUCTIONS:

1. Preheat oven to 400°F (200°C or gas mark 6).

2. Coat pork tenderloin with yellow mustard. Combine garlic powder, salt, and pepper. Evenly coat pork tenderloin with spice mixture.

3. Place pork in a large casserole dish and allow to rest for 20 to 30 minutes at room temperature.

4. Bake for 25 to 35 minutes or until the center has reached the desired temperature (a minimum of 145°F [63°C] for medium-rare, up to 160°F [71°C] for well done).

5. Baste pork in pan juices from the casserole dish and allow to rest for at least 5 minutes prior to slicing for service. Once sliced, baste each serving in remaining pan juices.

6. While pork is cooking/resting, boil turnips in a large pot of water for about 40 minutes or until tender.

7. Using a colander, drain turnips and allow to cool until steam is no longer visible to ensure excess moisture has evaporated. This will prevent the mash from becoming watery. Place cooled turnips into a food processor or large bowl for mashing or hand blending.

8. Heat olive oil and sage in a pan over medium heat for 2 to 3 minutes. Carefully drizzle hot oil and sage over turnips. Blend with a food processor or hand blender or manually mash to desired consistency. Season with salt to taste and serve.

NUTRITION FACTS:

Full Recipe: 1,133 calories, 42.7 g fat, 34.4 g total carbs, 10 g fiber (24.41 g net carbs), 147.8 g protein
Per Serving: 283 calories, 10.7 g fat, 8.6 g total carbs, 2.5 g fiber (6.10 g net carbs), 36.9 g protein

Slow Cooker Pot Roast

YIELD: 10 servings
SERVING SIZE: 3 to 4 ounces of meat (85 to 115 g) and ¹⁄₁₀ of the vegetables

PREP TIME: 10 minutes
COOK TIME: 8 to 10 hours
TOTAL TIME: 8 hours 10 minutes to 10 hours 10 minutes

A twist on a classic pot roast, here traditional ingredients are swapped for lower carb alternatives. Radishes and turnips are tasty substitutes for starchy carrots and potatoes in this dish.

INGREDIENTS:

1 teaspoon avocado oil or cooking fat of your choice

3 pounds (1.4 kg) boneless beef chuck roast

1 teaspoon salt

¼ teaspoon ground black pepper

1 medium onion, chopped

2 medium stalks celery, chopped

4 medium turnips, peeled and cubed

1 bunch radishes, stems removed

2 cloves garlic, minced

1 cup (235 ml) beef broth

1 bay leaf

INSTRUCTIONS:

1. Heat avocado oil over medium-high heat in a large skillet. Season beef with salt and pepper. Transfer beef to hot pan and brown on all sides.

2. Transfer browned beef to a large slow cooker. Add remaining ingredients around and on top of beef.

3. Place lid on slow cooker and cook on low for 8 to 10 hours. Remove bay leaf before serving.

NUTRITION FACTS:

Full Recipe: 2,097 calories, 83 g fat, 53.7 g total carbs, 14.9 g fiber (38.77 g net carbs), 289 g protein
Per Serving: 210 calories, 8.3 g fat, 5.4 g total carbs, 1.5 g fiber (3.88 g net carbs), 29 g protein

Tex-Mex Meatloaf

YIELD: 8 servings
SERVING SIZE: 1 slice

PREP TIME: 10 minutes
COOK TIME: 1 hour

TOTAL TIME: 1 hour 10 minutes

This Tex-Mex meatloaf delivers a spicy kick to a comfort food classic. Meatloaf is always a hit at dinner, and the leftovers are great meal prep material for weekday lunches!

SPECIAL DIET CONSIDERATIONS: Contains nuts and egg.

INGREDIENTS:

1 pound (455 g) lean ground beef

1 pound (455 g) ground pork

1 can (10 ounces, or 280 g) of Ro-Tel diced tomatoes and green chilies, or 10 ounces (280 g) fresh diced tomatoes and green chilies

1 jalapeño, diced

1 egg

¼ medium onion, diced

½ cup (56 g) almond four

1 teaspoon ground black pepper

1 teaspoon garlic powder

1 teaspoon salt

INSTRUCTIONS:

1. Preheat oven to 350°F (180°C or gas mark 4).

2. Combine all ingredients thoroughly in a large bowl.

3. Press meat mixture into a lightly greased 5 × 9-inch (13 × 23 cm) loaf pan. Alternatively, form into a 5 × 9-inch (13 × 23 cm) loaf shape on a greased baking dish.

4. Bake for 1 hour or until meatloaf reaches an internal temperature of 160°F (71°C). Let rest for 5 minutes before slicing. Slice into 8 even pieces. Serve with salsa and fresh salad.

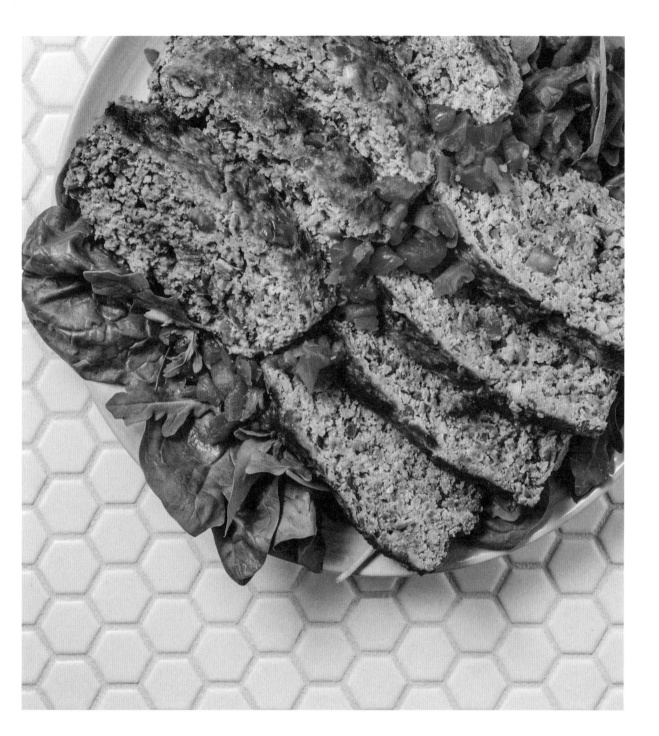

NUTRITION FACTS: **Full Recipe:** 2,817 calories, 180.5 g fat, 30 g total carbs, 10 g fiber (19.95 g net carbs), 264.1 g protein
Per Serving: 352.1 calories, 22.6 g fat, 3.7 g total carbs, 1.3 g fiber (2.49 g net carbs), 33 g protein

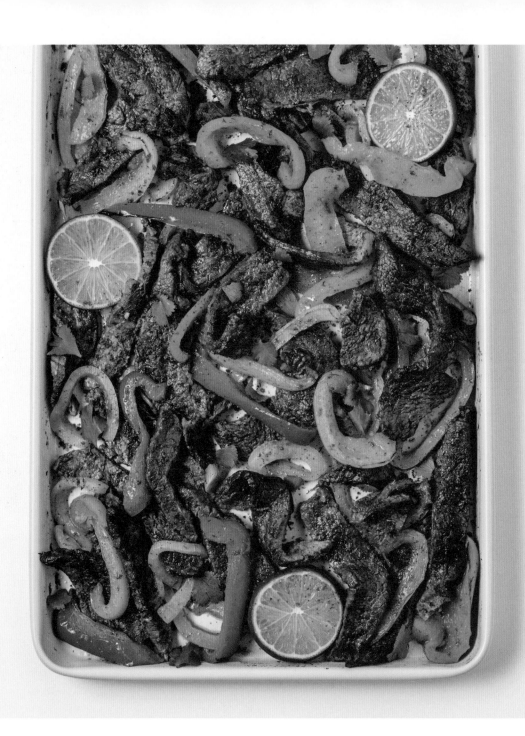

NUTRITION FACTS: **Full Recipe:** 2,056 calories, 96.4 g fat, 25.4 g carbs, 7.8 g fiber (17.62 g net carbs), 275 g protein
Per Serving: 343 calories, 16 g fat, 4.2 g total carbs, 1.3 g fiber (2.94 g net carbs), 45.8 g protein

Easy Sheet Pan Fajitas

YIELD: 6 servings
SERVING SIZE: ⅙ of the recipe

PREP TIME: 10 minutes
COOK TIME: 15 minutes

TOTAL TIME: 25 minutes

On busy nights when spending time in the kitchen feels nearly impossible, sheet pan meals are my go-to! What's not to love about tossing ingredients together on a pan and letting the oven do all the work while you handle other things? These fajitas are easy, healthy, and ready faster than a pizza delivery.

INGREDIENTS:

2 pounds (900 g) flank or skirt steak

¼ cup (60 ml) avocado oil

2 tablespoons (28 ml) freshly squeezed lime juice

¼ cup (4 g) minced cilantro

2 bell peppers, sliced

¼ medium onion, thinly sliced

½ teaspoon salt

¼ teaspoon chili powder

¼ teaspoon lime zest

INSTRUCTIONS:

1. Preheat oven to 425°F (220°C or gas mark 7) and set aside a large sheet pan.

2. Cut against the grain of the steak to make ¼ inch (6 mm)–thick strips of meat. Place in a large zipper lock bag. Add avocado oil, lime juice, cilantro, bell peppers, and onion to the bag and marinate at room temperature for approximately 5 minutes.

3. Using tongs, remove ingredients from the bag and spread across sheet pan in a single layer. Discard marinade and bag.

4. Place sheet pan in oven to cook for 10 minutes. Remove from oven and carefully toss ingredients on the sheet pan using tongs.

5. Set oven to broil on high heat. Place sheet pan back into the oven and broil for an additional 5 minutes.

6. Combine salt, chili powder, and lime zest. Remove fajitas from oven and sprinkle salt mixture evenly over the top to taste. Serve immediately.

NOTE: The fajitas can be enjoyed alone or served with lettuce leaf "tortillas."

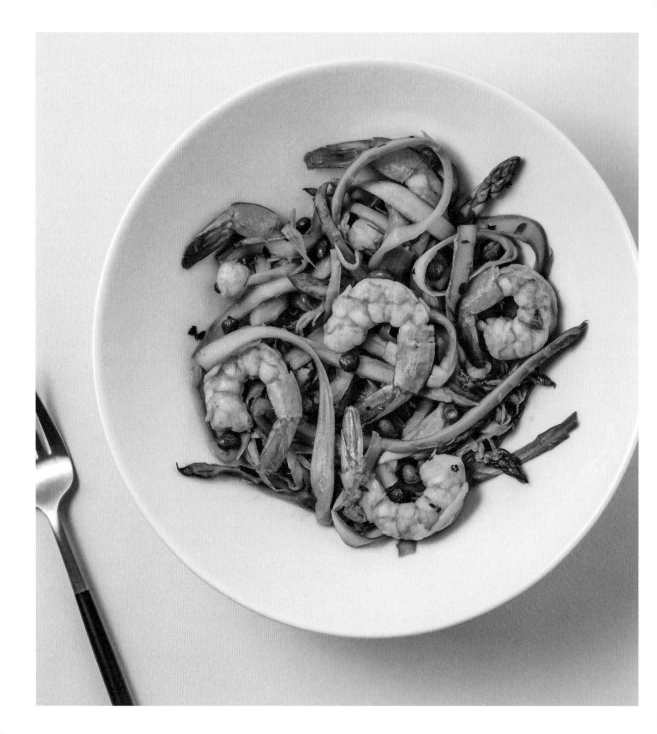

NUTRITION FACTS: **Full Recipe:** 372 calories, 16.8 g fat, 18 g total carbs, 8.7 g fiber (9.34 g net carbs), 41 g protein
Per Serving: 186 calories, 8.4 g fat, 9 g total carbs, 4.3 g fiber (4.67 g net carbs), 20.6 g protein

Shrimp with Asparagus Noodles

YIELD: 2 servings
SERVING SIZE: half of the recipe

PREP TIME: 5 minutes
COOK TIME: 5 minutes

TOTAL TIME: 10 minutes

Asparagus is delicious no matter the preparation, but have you ever thought to use it as noodles? Thinly shaving the asparagus lengthwise produces flavorful ribbons that can be used as a pasta or noodle substitute in any dish.

INGREDIENTS:

20 large spears asparagus

1 tablespoon (15 ml) olive oil or cooking fat of choice

8 ounces (225 g) raw shrimp, cleaned and deveined

1 tablespoon (9 g) capers

1 teaspoon fresh, minced basil

1 teaspoon minced anchovies or anchovy paste

INSTRUCTIONS:

1. Using a sharp vegetable peeler or mandoline, carefully shave asparagus lengthwise into thin strips. If using a vegetable peeler, it helps to place asparagus along the edge of a flat cutting board to access more surface area of the vegetable. Set shaved asparagus aside.

2. In a large frying pan with fitted lid, heat olive oil over low medium heat. Add shrimp to pan.

3. When shrimp begins to turn opaque on the bottom, add asparagus, capers, basil, and anchovies. Toss with tongs to distribute ingredients and place lid over pan until shrimp is fully cooked or completely opaque. Shrimp cooks quickly; it will take around 4 to 5 minutes total.

4. Remove lid from pan when shrimp is fully cooked and transfer contents of the pan to serving dishes. Serve immediately.

NOTE: If you have an allergy to shellfish, shrimp can be replaced with another protein source, such as chicken, beef, pork, or egg, though cooking time will require adjustment

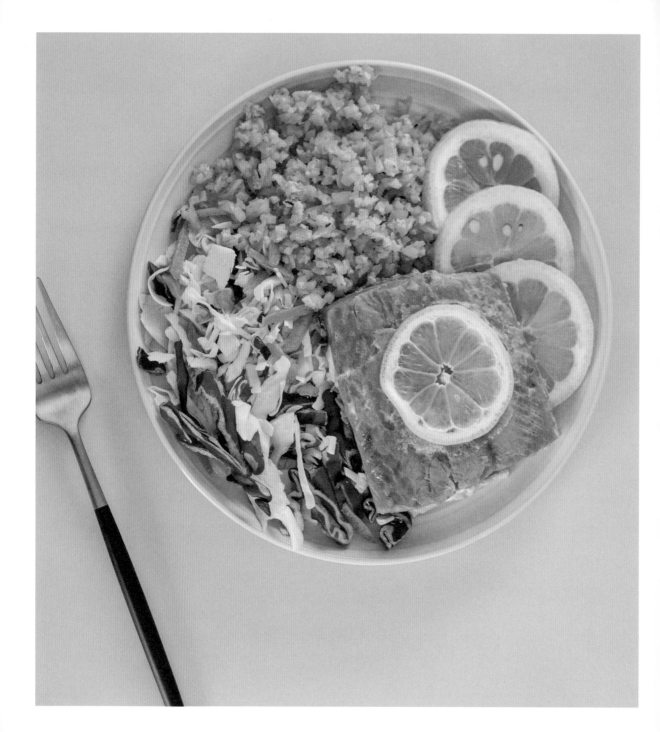

NUTRITION FACTS: **Full Recipe:** 1,405 calories, 62.3 g fat, 52.4 g total carbs, 19.3 g fiber (33.09 g net carbs), 162.1 g protein
Per Serving: 351 calories, 15.6 g fat, 13.1 g total carbs, 4.8 g fiber (8.27 g net carbs), 40.5 g protein

Mediterranean Salmon and Rice

YIELD: 4 servings
SERVING SIZE: 1 salmon fillet and
   ¼ of the cauliflower rice

PREP TIME: 10 minutes
COOK TIME: 20 minutes
TOTAL TIME: 30 minutes

Brimming with omega-3s, protein, selenium, potassium, B-vitamins, vitamin C, choline, folate, magnesium, and more, this dish is an absolute nutritional powerhouse! It's also quick and easy to prepare—who said healthy eating has to be hard?

INGREDIENTS:

nonstick cooking spray

1 large head cauliflower, riced

2 cloves garlic, minced

¼ medium onion, minced

1 teaspoon ground turmeric

½ teaspoon dried thyme

1 tablespoon (15 ml) olive oil

2 tablespoons (28 ml) chicken broth

salt to taste

ground black pepper to taste

4 boneless salmon fillets (5 ounces, or 140 g each)

1 small lemon, sliced

INSTRUCTIONS:

1. Preheat oven to 375°F (190°C or gas mark 5).

2. Spray a 9 × 11-inch (23 × 28 cm) casserole dish with small amount of nonstick cooking spray.

3. Combine cauliflower, garlic, onion, turmeric, thyme, olive oil, chicken broth, salt, and pepper. Transfer mixture to casserole dish and spread in an even layer.

4. Place salmon fillets on top of cauliflower mixture. Top with lemon slices and cover dish with foil.

5. Bake for 15 to 20 minutes or until salmon is completely cooked through. Carefully remove foil and serve.

Smoked Salmon Boats

YIELD: 4 servings (16 lettuce boats)
SERVING SIZE: 4 lettuce boats

PREP TIME: 15 minutes
TOTAL TIME: 15 minutes

I love lettuce boats for the simplicity of the preparation and the unique combinations that yield delicious results. This recipe is so simple, it doesn't require any cooking at all! Rotisserie chicken, canned tuna, or shaved turkey from the deli all make fantastic no-cook proteins that can be used in a similar fashion.

INGREDIENTS:

16 Belgian endive, romaine, or Bibb lettuce leaves, individually separated

1 avocado, chopped

½ teaspoon lemon juice

1 pound (455 g) smoked salmon, chopped

¼ cup (34 g) capers

2 tablespoons (8 g) fresh dill

salt to taste

INSTRUCTIONS:

1. Wash and dry lettuce leaves.

2. Toss avocado in lemon juice.

3. Combine avocado, salmon, and capers. Divide mixture on top of lettuce leaves.

4. Garnish with dill and salt to taste. Serve immediately.

NOTE: To suit your preferences, any sturdy lettuce leaf can be used in this recipe in place of endive, Romaine, or Bibb.

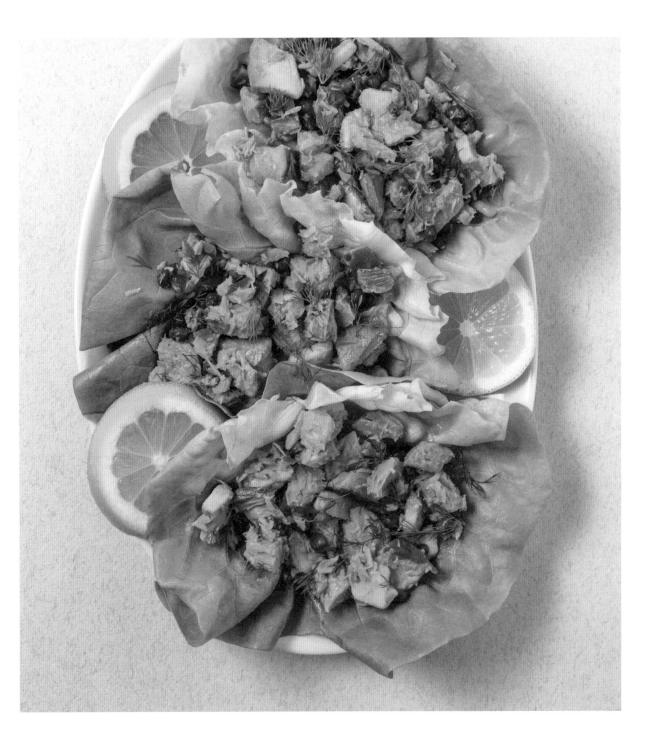

NUTRITION FACTS: **Full Recipe:** 783.2 calories, 41.1 g fat, 16.6 g total carbs, 11.7 g fiber (4.90 g net carbs), 88.1 g protein
Per Serving: 196 calories, 10.3 g fat, 4.2 g total carbs, 2.9 g fiber (1.22 g net carbs), 22 g protein

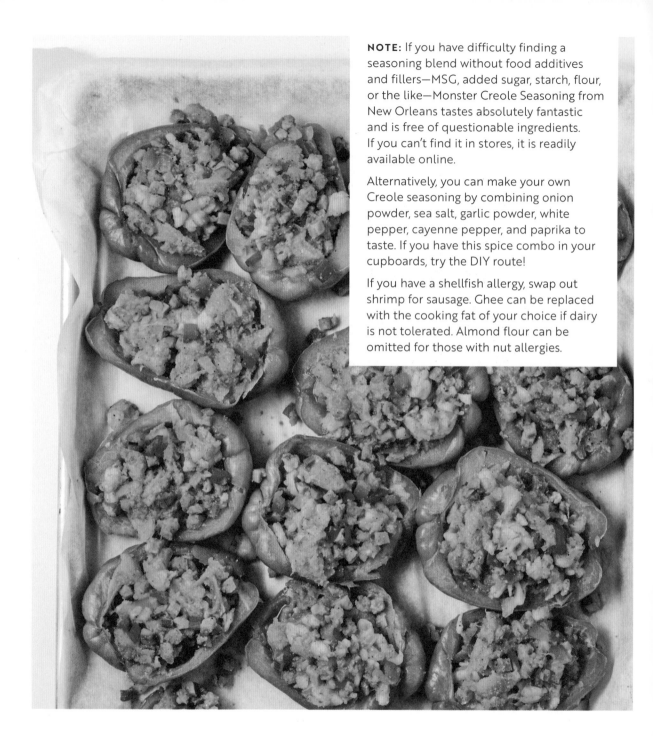

NOTE: If you have difficulty finding a seasoning blend without food additives and fillers—MSG, added sugar, starch, flour, or the like—Monster Creole Seasoning from New Orleans tastes absolutely fantastic and is free of questionable ingredients. If you can't find it in stores, it is readily available online.

Alternatively, you can make your own Creole seasoning by combining onion powder, sea salt, garlic powder, white pepper, cayenne pepper, and paprika to taste. If you have this spice combo in your cupboards, try the DIY route!

If you have a shellfish allergy, swap out shrimp for sausage. Ghee can be replaced with the cooking fat of your choice if dairy is not tolerated. Almond flour can be omitted for those with nut allergies.

NUTRITION FACTS: **Full Recipe:** 1,104 calories, 35.3 g fat, 106.2 g total carbs, 32.9 g fiber (73.2 g net carbs), 122.7 g protein
Per Serving: 138 calories, 4.4 g fat, 13.3 g total carbs, 4.1 g fiber (9.16 g net carbs), 15.3 g protein

Stuffed Mirlitons

YIELD: 8 servings
SERVING SIZE: 2 stuffed mirlitons

PREP TIME: 20 minutes
COOK TIME: 1 hour 10 minutes
TOTAL TIME: 1 hour 30 minutes

Never heard of a mirliton? Don't feel bad; these small, green squash are called something different in every part of the word. Mirliton, chayote squash, pear squash, cho-cho, chochoute, choko—whatever you call it, this fruit/veggie is surprisingly low in carbohydrates, is packed with micronutrients, and makes a killer substitute for potatoes, apples, and even noodles!

Hailing from Louisiana, stuffed mirlitons are a special comfort food treat that is often prepared for holiday gatherings. This keto-compatible version of the traditional side dish is a bit labor intensive, but it's undoubtedly worth the extra effort.

SPECIAL DIET CONSIDERATIONS: Contains shellfish, nuts, and dairy.

INGREDIENTS:

8 mirlitons (chayote squash)

1 teaspoon ghee or cooking fat of choice

¼ medium onion, minced

2 stalks celery, diced

¼ medium red bell pepper, diced

1 pound (455 g) fresh shrimp, peeled and chopped

½ pound (225 g) uncured ham, chopped

2 tablespoons (22 g) Creole seasoning

¼ cup (28 g) almond meal or flour

INSTRUCTIONS:

1. Boil mirlitons in a large stock pot filled with water about 40 minutes, until tender. Remove mirlitons from water and let rest until cool to the touch.

2. Cut mirlitons in half lengthwise and discard seeds. Gently scoop flesh from each half and reserve in a fine mesh colander, leaving the skin with a ¼-inch (6 mm) border of squash intact. Mash the flesh in the colander, allowing water to drip off into the sink. Invert the skins on paper towels to drain off excess moisture.

3. Preheat oven to 300°F (150°C or gas mark 2) and line a large sheet pan with parchment paper.

4. Discard water from the stockpot and melt ghee over medium heat. Add onion, celery, and red bell pepper. Cook until onion becomes translucent. Stir in shrimp and ham. Cook until shrimp is no longer translucent.

5. Remove stockpot from heat. Stir in reserved mirliton flesh, Creole seasoning, and almond meal until thoroughly combined.

6. Generously stuff each mirliton skin with shrimp mixture. Place stuffing-side up on the parchment paper-lined sheet pan or a casserole dish. Cover mirlitons with foil and bake for 20 minutes. Serve alone or as a side dish.

Meatza

YIELD: 4 servings (8 slices)
SERVING SIZE: 2 slices

PREP TIME: 10 minutes
COOK TIME: 30 minutes

TOTAL TIME: 40 minutes

Craving pizza? Don't stoop to eating the toppings of a carb-loaded delivery and tossing out the crust. Make your own keto-compatible pizza! Load it up with your favorite low-carb pizza toppings or try out my favorites below.

SPECIAL DIET CONSIDERATIONS: The recipe as written is dairy-free. If dairy is well tolerated, feel free to replace nutritional yeast with shredded, low-moisture mozzarella cheese.

INGREDIENTS:

1 pound (455 g) ground turkey, chicken, or lean beef

½ cup (30 g) nutritional yeast, divided

1 egg

1 tablespoon (3 g) dried or (4 g) fresh oregano

½ teaspoon garlic powder

¼ cup (60 ml) Sugar-free Spaghetti Sauce (see page 247)

¼ medium red onion, sliced

½ cup (10 g) arugula

¼ cup (25 g) sliced black olives

INSTRUCTIONS:

1. Preheat oven to 400°F (200°C or gas mark 6) and line a large baking pan with parchment paper.

2. Combine turkey, ¼ cup (15 g) of nutritional yeast, egg, oregano, and garlic powder.

3. Spread mixture onto the parchment paper and press into an even ¼-inch (6 mm) thick layer.

4. Bake for 20 minutes or until cooked through.

5. Carefully remove from oven and drain any accumulated grease.

6. Spread sauce evenly over the cooked turkey crust.

7. Garnish with red onion, arugula, olives, and remaining ¼ cup (15 g) of nutritional yeast.

8. Bake for an additional 10 minutes. Remove from oven and let cool 5 to 10 minutes prior to slicing. Cut into 8 even pieces.

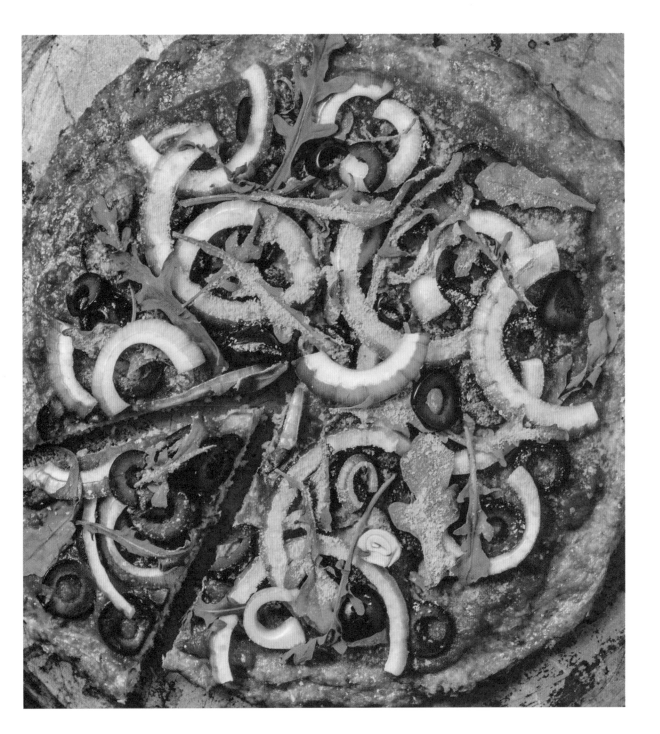

NUTRITION FACTS: **Full Recipe:** 1,503 calories, 91.5 g fat, 24.5 g total carbs, 10.4 g fiber (14.10 g net carbs), 145.6 g protein
Per Serving: 376 calories, 22.9 g fat, 6.1 g total carbs, 2.6 g fiber (3.52 g net carbs), 36.4 g protein

Dirty Rice

YIELD: 6 servings
SERVING SIZE: ⅙ of the recipe
  (approx. 1½ cups [300 g])

PREP TIME: 10 minutes
COOK TIME: 20 minutes
TOTAL TIME: 30 minutes

With a name like *dirty rice*, you might be surprised by just how good this dish tastes. Rich, aromatic, and packed with vitamins and minerals, this classic one-pot dish is guaranteed to satisfy your hunger and nourish your body.

INGREDIENTS:

1 pound (455 g) ground pork or beef

¼ medium onion, diced

1 rib celery, chopped

½ green bell pepper, diced

1 large head cauliflower, riced

¼ cup (60 ml) chicken stock

1 teaspoon paprika

1 teaspoon garlic powder

½ teaspoon cayenne pepper

½ teaspoon dried thyme

4 ounces (115 g) chicken livers, trimmed of fat and membrane and minced

salt to taste

ground black pepper to taste

INSTRUCTIONS:

1. Brown pork over medium-high heat in a large skillet. Break meat down with a utensil to yield small, crumbly pieces.

2. When meat is no longer pink, add onion, celery, bell pepper, and cauliflower to the pan. Cook for 2 to 3 minutes.

3. Add chicken stock, paprika, garlic powder, cayenne, and thyme. Mix thoroughly and bring to a boil. Reduce to a simmer.

4. Add chicken livers and cook for 5 to 6 minutes or until liquid has evaporated and liver has fully cooked. Season with salt and pepper to taste and serve.

NUTRITION FACTS:

Full Recipe: 1,758 calories, 42 g total carbs, 15.7 g fiber (26.16 g net carbs), 165 g protein
Per Serving: 293 calories, 7 g total carbs, 2.6 g fiber (4.36 g net carbs), 27.5 g protein

Sugar-Free Spaghetti Sauce

YIELD: 14 servings (3½ cups [825 ml])
SERVING SIZE: ¼ cup (60 ml)

PREP TIME: 5 minutes
COOK TIME: 30 minutes
TOTAL TIME: 35 minutes

Due to added sugar and starchy thickeners, sauces and condiments are yet another group of ingredients that often yield surprisingly high carb counts. Jarred tomato and marinara sauces are no exception. Preparing your own spaghetti sauce gives you control over the carb content and flavor profile, and it always tastes so much better!

INGREDIENTS:

¼ cup (60 ml) extra virgin olive oil

5 cloves garlic, minced

1 can (28 ounces, or 785 g) of whole peeled tomatoes, or prepare 2 pounds (900 g) fresh, peeled tomatoes

1 cup (235 ml) water

½ teaspoon dried oregano

½ teaspoon dried basil

salt to taste

INSTRUCTIONS:

1. In a large saucepan, heat olive oil over medium-low heat. Add garlic to oil. Gently stir and simmer for about 1 minute.

2. Smash whole tomatoes with a utensil while garlic simmers. Add tomatoes, 1 cup (235 ml) of water, oregano, and basil to the saucepan.

3. Reduce heat to low and simmer for 15 to 20 minutes, stirring occasionally. Taste sauce and season with salt to taste.

4. Serve immediately or store refrigerated in airtight glass jars.

NOTE: Canned tomatoes were used in this recipe for ease of preparation, but you can use fresh tomatoes if you prefer! Simply blanch tomatoes in a large stockpot of boiling water for several minutes, allow to cool, and gently remove skin. Now they're ready to use!

Feel free to experiment with different flavors to re-create your favorite sauces.

Serve on vegetable noodles, low-carb pizza (like the Meatza on page 244), as a shakshuka base, or simply as a condiment.

NUTRITION FACTS:

Full Recipe: 665 calories, 54 g fat, 38 g total carbs, 7.2 g fiber (30.84 g net carbs), 7.6 g protein
Per Serving: 48 calories, 3.9 g fat, 2.7 g total carbs, 0.5 g fiber (2.20 g net carbs), 0.5 g protein

Taco Seasoning

YIELD: 12 tablespoons (103 g)
SERVING SIZE: 1 tablespoon (6 g)

PREP TIME: 5 minutes
TOTAL TIME: 5 minutes

As you begin to reduce carbohydrates in your diet, you may be surprised by the carb counts in many premade seasoning packets and dressings. My biggest shock of all was taco seasoning packets, which are loaded with sugars, starches, and other food additives. Whipping up a batch of homemade taco seasoning is a great way to preserve the flavor and dramatically reduce the carb content of taco night!

INGREDIENTS:

¼ cup (24 g) ground cumin

¼ cup (30 g) chili powder

2 tablespoons (18 g) garlic powder

1 tablespoon (7 g) onion powder

1 tablespoon (18 g) salt

1 teaspoon paprika

1 teaspoon dried oregano

INSTRUCTIONS:

Taco Seasoning

1. In a glass mason jar with a fitted lid, combine cumin, chili powder, garlic powder, onion powder, salt, paprika, and oregano.

2. Screw on lid and store in a spice cabinet to use as needed.

For Use in Taco Meat Preparation

1. Brown meat of choice in a large skillet and remove excess rendered fat. Add 1 tablespoon (6 g) of prepared taco seasoning per pound (455 g) of meat, add ¾ cup (175 ml) water, stir evenly, and bring to a boil. Reduce heat and simmer for 2 to 3 minutes.

2. Serve as taco filling, in taco salad, or in burrito bowls.

NOTE: Use 1 tablespoon (6 g) of seasoning to replace 1 taco seasoning packet.

Use 1 tablespoon (6 g) of seasoning per pound (455 g) of meat; adjust to taste.

NUTRITION FACTS:

Full Recipe: 277 calories, 10.5 g fat, 48 g total carbs, 17.7 g fiber (30.34 g net carbs), 13 g protein
Per Serving: 23 calories, 0.9 g fat, 4 g total carbs, 1.5 g fiber (2.53 g net carbs), 1.1 g protein

DIY Mayo

YIELD: 16 servings (approx. 1 cup [240 g] total)
SERVING SIZE: 1 tablespoon (15 g)

PREP TIME: 5 minutes
TOTAL TIME: 5 minutes

Some manufacturers are starting to use more health-minded ingredients to make mayonnaise, but most commercially available brands aren't. If you are having trouble finding mayonnaise made with ingredients you trust, this easy DIY Mayo recipe will give you the flexibility to source your own quality ingredients. And of course, it tastes a million times better than store-bought mayo!

INGREDIENTS:

2 egg yolks

1 tablespoon (15 ml) lemon juice

1 tablespoon (15 ml) apple cider vinegar

¼ teaspoon salt

1 teaspoon Dijon mustard

¾ cup (175 ml) avocado oil

INSTRUCTIONS:

Using an Immersion Blender:

1. Place ingredients in a 16-ounce (473 ml) wide-mouth mason jar in this order: egg, lemon juice, apple cider vinegar, salt, mustard, avocado oil.

2. Place an immersion hand blender in, all the way to the bottom of the jar, and switch the tool on to the highest speed, keeping blender stationary for 10 to 15 seconds.

3. Once the emulsion begins to form, move the blender up and down to incorporate all the ingredients.

4. Cover with lid and refrigerate until ready to use. Store in refrigerator up to 1 week.

NOTE: I enjoy using an immersion blender to prevent dirtying multiple dishes. Less clean up! But if you don't have an immersion blender, you can prepare this recipe in a traditional blender or food processor by changing the order of the steps around: Place all ingredients except the oil into a standard blender or food processor and pulse until the mixture becomes frothy. With the blender running, very slowly drizzle oil in until the emulsion forms and all ingredients have been incorporated. Transfer to a glass storage container and refrigerate until needed.

NUTRITION FACTS:

Full Recipe: 1,560 calories, 172 g fat, 2.6 g total carbs, 0.2 g fiber (2.35 g net carbs), 5.5 g protein
Per Serving: 97.5 calories, 10.8 g fat, 0.2 g total carbs, 0 g fiber (0.2 g net carbs), 0.3 g protein

Resources

Macronutrient and Calorie Tracker
cronometer.com

Macronutrient Calculator
ketogasm.com/keto-calculator

United States Department of Agriculture (USDA) Food Composition Databases
ndb.nal.usda.gov/ndb

References

Chapter 1

1. Westman, E. C., J. Mavropoulos, W. S. Yancy, and J. S. Volek. "A Review of Low-Carbohydrate Ketogenic Diets." *Current Atherosclerosis Reports* 5, no. 6 (November 2003):476–483.

2. Kaleta, C., L. F. de Figueiredo, S. Werner, R. Guthke, M. Ristow, and S. Schuster. "*In Silico* Evidence for Gluconeogenesis from Fatty Acids in Humans." *PLOS Computational Biology* 7, no. 7 (July 2011). doi.org /10.1371/journal.pcbi.1002116.

   Phinney, S. D. "Ketogenic Diets and Physical Performance." *Nutrition and Metabolism* 1, no. 1 (August 2004). doi:10.1186/1743-7075-1-2.

3. Phinney, "Ketogenic Diets," 2004.

4. Roehl, K., and S. L. Sewak. "Practice Paper of the Academy of Nutrition and Dietetics: Classic and Modified Ketogenic Diets for Treatment of Epilepsy." *Journal of the Academy of Nutrition and Dietetics* 117, no. 8 (August 2017): 1279–1292. doi:10.1016/j.jand.2017.06.006.

5. Berger, A. *The Alzheimer's Antidote: Using a Low-Carb, High-Fat Diet to Fight Alzheimer's Disease, Memory Loss, and Cognitive Decline*. White River Junction, VT: Chelsea Green Publishing, 2017.

6. Koppel, S. J., and R. H. Swerdlow. "Neuroketotherapeutics: A Modern Review of a Century-Old Therapy." *Neurochemistry International* 117 (July 2018): 114–125. doi:10.1016 /j.neuint.2017.05.019.

7. Hussain, T. A., T. C. Mathew, A. A. Dashti, S. Asfar, N. Al-Zaid, and H. M Dashti. "Applied Nutritional Investigation: Effect of Low-Calorie versus Low-Carbohydrate Ketogenic Diet in Type 2 Diabetes." *Nutrition* 28, no.10 (October 2012): 1016–1021. doi:10.1016 /j.nut.2012.01.016.

8. Banting, W. "Letter on Corpulence, Addressed to the Public." 1863. *Obesity Research* 1, no. 2 (March 1993): 153–163.

9. Atkins, R. C. *Dr. Atkins' Diet Revolution*. New York: Bantam Books Publishing, 1973.

   Atkins, R. C. *Atkins for Life: The Complete Diet for Permanent Weight Loss and Good Health*. London: Macmillan Publishers, 2003.

10. Cordain, L. *The Paleo Diet Revised: Lose Weight and Get Healthy by Eating the Foods You Were Designed to Eat.* Boston: Houghton Mifflin Harcourt, 2010.

11. Chang, J., and S. R. Kashyap. "The Protein-Sparing Modified Fast for Obese Patients with Type 2 Diabetes: What to Expect." *Cleveland Clinical Journal of Medicine* 81, no. 9 (September 2014): 557–565.

Chapter 2

1. Volek, J. S., and S .D. Phinney, *The Art and Science of Low Carbohydrate Performance.* Miami: Beyond Obesity LLC, 2012.

2. Health Canada. "Proposed Policy: Definition and Energy Value for Dietary Fibre." 2010. Government of Canada Retrieved from www.canada.ca/en/health-canada/services/food-nutrition/public-involvement-partnerships/proposed-policy-definition-energy-value-dietary-fibre/consultation.html.

3. Jeukendrup, A. E. "Carbohydrate Feeding during Exercise." *European Journal of Sport Science* 8, no. 2 (March 2008): 77–86. doi:10.1080/17461390801918971.

4. Ljubicic, M., M. M. Saric, I. Rumbak, I. C. Baric, D. Komes, Z. Satalic, and R. P. F. Guiné. "Knowledge about Dietary Fibre and Its Health Benefits: A Cross-Sectional Survey of 2,536 Residents from across Croatia." *Medical Hypotheses* 105 (August 2017): 25–31. doi:10.1016/j.mehy.2017.06.019.

5. Gross, L. S., L. Li, E. S. Ford, and S. Liu. "Increased Consumption of Refined Carbohydrates and the Epidemic of Type 2 Diabetes in the United States: An Ecologic Assessment." *The American Journal of Clinical Nutrition* 79, no. 5 (May 2004): 774–779.

6. Ibid.

7. Gropper, S. S., J. L. Smith, and T. P. Carr. *Advanced Nutrition and Human Metabolism*, 7th edition. Boston: Cengage Learning, 2018.

8. Centers for Disease Control and Prevention. "National Diabetes Statistics Report." 2017. Retrieved from www.cdc.gov/diabetes/data/statistics/statistics-report.html.

9. Ibid.

10. Badri, N. W., S. W. Flatt, H. S. Barkai, B. Pakiz, D. D. Heath, et al. "Insulin Resistance Improves More in Women than in Men in Association with a Weight Loss Intervention." *Journal of Obesity and Weight Loss Therapy* 8, no. 1 (February 2019): 365. doi:10.4172/2165-7904.1000365.

11. Groper et al., 2018.

12. Taha, A. Y., Cheon, Y., Faurot, K. F., MacIntosh, B., Majchrzak-Hong, S. F., Mann, J. D., et al. "Dietary Omega-6 Fatty Acid Lowering Increases Bioavailability of Omega-3 Polyunsaturated Fatty Acids in Human Plasma Lipid Pools." *Prostaglandins, Leukotrienes and Essential Fatty Acids* 90, no. 5 (May 2014): 151–157. doi:10.1016/j.plefa.2014.02.003.

13. Westman, E. C., J. Mavropoulos, W. S. Yancy, and J. S. Volek. "A Review of Low-Carbohydrate Ketogenic Diets." *Current Atherosclerosis Reports* 5, no. 6 (November 2003): 476–483.

14. Institute of Medicine. *Dietary Reference Intakes for Energy, Carbohydrate, Fiber, Fat, Fatty Acids, Cholesterol, Protein, and Amino Acids.* Washington, DC: The National Academies Press, 2005.

15. Gropper et al., 2018.

16. Taha et al., 2014.

17. Sears, B., and M. Perry. "The Role of Fatty Acids in Insulin Resistance." *Lipids in Health and Disease* 14 (2015): 121. doi:10.1186/s12944-015-0123-1.

Taha et al., 2014.

18. Taha et al., 2014.

19. M. A. Veldhorst, M. S. Westerterp-Plantenga, and K. R. Westerterp. "Gluconeogenesis and Energy Expenditure After a High-Protein, Carbohydrate-Free Diet." *The American Journal of Clinical Nutrition* 90, no. 3 (September 2009): 519–526. doi:10.3945/ajcn.2009.27834.

20. Volek and Phinney, 2012.

21. Das, S., and T. F. Smith. "Identifying Nature's Protein Lego Set." *Advances in Protein Chemistry* 54 (2000): 159–183.

22. Gropper et al., 2018.

23. Arentson-Lantz, E., S. Clairmont, D. Paddon-Jones, A. Tremblay, and R. Elango. "Protein: A Nutrient in Focus." *Applied Physiology, Nutrition and Metabolism* 40, no. 8 (August 2015): 755–761. doi.org/10.1139/apnm-2014-0530.

Rodriguez, N. R., and S. L. Miller. "Effective Translation of Current Dietary Guidance: Understanding and Communicating the Concepts of Minimal and Optimal Levels of Dietary Protein." *American Journal of Clinical Nutrition* 101, no. 6 (April 2015): 1353S–1358S. doi.org/10.3945/ajcn.114.084095.

24. Volek and Phinney, 2012.

25. Rodriguez et al., 2015

Leaf and Antonio, 2017.

26. Chambers, L., K. McCrickerd, and M. R. Yeomans. "Optimising Foods for Satiety." *Trends in Food Science and Technology* 41, no. 2 (February 2015): 149–160. doi.org/10.1016/j.tifs.2014.10.007.

27. Institute of Medicine, 2005.

28. Ibid.

29. Leaf, A., and J. Antonio. "The Effects of Overfeeding on Body Composition: The Role of Macronutrient Composition—A Narrative Review." *International Journal of Exercise Science* 10, no. 8 (December 2017): 1275–1296.

30. Westman et al., 2003.

31. Veldhorst et al., 2009.

32. Volek and Phinney, 2012.

Diet Doctor. Low-Carb Living [Video File]. (December 6, 2011). Retrieved from www.dietdoctor.com/low-carb-living.

Giezenaar, C., K. Lange, T. Hausken, K. L. Jones, M. Horowitz, I. Chapman, and S. Soenen. "Acute Effects of Substitution, and Addition, of Carbohydrates and Fat to Protein on Gastric Emptying, Blood Glucose, Gut Hormones, Appetite, and Energy Intake." *Nutrients* 10, no. 10 (October 2018): pii: E1451. doi:10.3390/nu10101451.

McDevitt, R. M., S. J. Bott, M. Harding, W. A. Coward, L. J. Bluck, and A. M. Prentice. "De Novo Lipogenesis during Controlled Overfeeding with Sucrose or Glucose in Lean and Obese Women." *American Journal of Clinical Nutrition* 74, no. 6 (December 2001): 737–746. doi.org/10.1093/ajcn/74.6.737.

Menke A., S. Casagrande, L. Geiss, and C.C. Cowie. "Prevalence of and Trends in Diabetes among Adults in the United States, 1988–2012." *JAMA* 314, no. 10 (September 2015):1021–1029. doi:10.1001/jama.2015.10029.

Chapter 3

1. McGuire, S. "Scientific Report of the 2015 Dietary Guidelines Advisory Committee." Washington, DC: U.S. Departments of Agriculture and Health and Human Services, 2015.

2. DiFeliceantonio, A. G., G. Coppin, L. Rigoux, S. Edwin Thanarajah, A. Dagher, M. Tittgemeyer, and D. M. Small. "Supra-Additive Effects of Combining Fat and Carbohydrate on Food Reward." *Cell Metabolism* 28, no. 1 (July 2018): 33–44.e3. doi:10.1016/j.cmet.2018.05.018.

3. Ibid.

4. Voigt, J.P., and H. Fink. "Serotonin Controlling Feeding and Satiety." *Behavioural Brain Research* 277 (January 2015): 14–31. doi:10.1016/j.bbr.2014.08.065.

5. Mauvais-Jarvis, F. "Sex Differences in Metabolic Homeostasis, Diabetes, and Obesity." *Biology of Sex Differences* 6, no. 1 (2015): 14. doi:10.1186/s13293-015-0033-y.

6. Ibid.

7. Phinney, S. D., E. S. Horton, E. A. Sims, J. S. Hanson, E. Danforth Jr., and B. M. LaGrange. "Capacity for Moderate Exercise in Obese Subjects After Adaptation to a Hypocaloric, Ketogenic Diet." *Journal of Clinical Investigation* 66, no. 5 (November 1980): 1152–1161.

McSwiney, F. T., B. Wardrop, P. N. Hyde, R. A. Lafountain, J. S. Volek, and L. Doyle. "Keto-Adaptation Enhances Exercise Performance and Body Composition Responses to Training in Endurance Athletes." *Metabolism: Clinical and Experimental* 81 (April 2018): 25–34. doi.org/10.1016/j.metabol.2017.10.010.

8. Volek, J. S., and S. D. Phinney. *The Art and Science of Low Carbohydrate Performance*. Miami: Beyond Obesity LLC, 2012.

9. Westman, E. C., J. Mavropoulos, W. S. Yancy, and J. S. Volek. "A Review of Low-Carbohydrate Ketogenic Diets." *Current Atherosclerosis Reports* 5, no. 6 (November 2003):476–483.

10. Fedorovich, S. V., P. P. Voronina, and T. V. Waseem. "Ketogenic Diet *versus* Ketoacidosis: What Determines the Influence of Ketone Bodies on Neurons?" *Neural Regeneration Research* 13, no. 12 (December 2018): 2060–2063. doi:10.4103/167305374.241442.

11. Ibid.

12. Gibson, A. A., R. V. Seimon, C. M. Lee, J. Ayre, J. Franklin, T. P. Markovic, I. D. Caterson, and A. Sainsbury. "Do Ketogenic Diets Really Suppress Appetite? A Systematic Review and Meta-Analysis." *Obesity Reviews* 16, no. 1 (November 2014): 64–76. doi.org/10.1111/obr.12230.

13. Nymo, S., S. R. Coutinho, J. Jorgensen, J. F. Rehfeld, H. Truby, B. Kulseng, and C. Martins. "Timeline of Changes in Appetite During Weight Loss with a Ketogenic Diet." *International Journal of Obesity* 41, no. 8 (August 2017): 1224–1231. doi:10.1038/ijo.2017.96.

Gibson et al., 2014.

14. López-Alarcón, M., O. Perichart-Perera, S. Flores-Huerta, P. Inda-Icaza, M. Rodríguez-Cruz, A. Armenta-Álvarez, M. T. Bram-Falcón, et al. "Excessive Refined Carbohydrates and Scarce Micronutrient Intakes Increase Inflammatory Mediators and Insulin Resistance in Prepubertal and Pubertal Obese Children Independently of Obesity." *Mediators of Inflammation* (2014): doi:10.1155/2014/849031.

Hawkins, M. A. W., N. G. Keirns, and Z. Helms. "Carbohydrates and Cognitive Function." *Current Opinion in Clinical Nutrition and Metabolic Care* 21, no. 4 (July 2018): 302–307. doi:10.1097/MCO.0000000000000471.

Delibasi, T., and E. Cakir. "Is Refined Carbohydrate Consumption Related to Allergic Diseases?" *Nutrition* 30, no. 4 (April 2014): 401–402. doi:10.1016/j.nut.2013.09.018.

15. Wright, C., and N. L. Simone. "Obesity and Tumor Growth: Inflammation, Immunity, and the Role of a Ketogenic Diet." *Current Opinion in Clinical Nutrition and Metabolic Care* 19, no. 4 (July 2016): 2949. doi:10.1097/MCO.0000000000000286.

Tedeschi, S. K., and K. H. Costenbader. "Is There a Role for Diet in the Therapy of Rheumatoid Arthritis?" *Current Rheumatology Reports* 18, no. 5 (May 2016): 23. doi:10.1007/s11926-016-0575-y.

16. Barrea, L., P. Marzullo, G. Muscogiuri, C. Di Somma, M. Scacchi, F. Orio, G. Aimaretti, et al. "Source and Amount of Carbohydrate in the Diet and Inflammation in Women with Polycystic Ovary Syndrome." *Nutrition Research Reviews* 31, no. 2 (December 2018): 291–301. doi:10.1017/S0954422418000136.

17. Bianchi, V. E. Review: "Weight Loss Is a Critical Factor to Reduce Inflammation." *Clinical Nutrition ESPEN* 28 (December 2018): 21–35. doi:10.1016/j.clnesp.2018.08.007.

18. Brietzke, E., R. B. Mansur, M. Subramaniapillai, V. Balanzá-Martínez, M. Vinberg, A. González-Pinto, J. D. Rosenblat, et al. "Ketogenic Diet as a Metabolic Therapy for Mood Disorders: Evidence and Developments." *Neuroscience and Biobehavioral Reviews* 94 (November 2018): 11–16. doi:10.1016/j.neubiorev.2018.07.020.

19. Cargill, K. *Food Cults: How Fads, Dogma, and Doctrine Influence Diet.* Lanham, MD: Rowman and Littlefield, 2016.

20. Ibid.

21. Christoph, M. J., N. Larson, K. C. Hootman, J. M. Miller, and D. Neumark-Sztainer. (2018). "Who Values Gluten-Free? Dietary Intake, Behaviors, and Sociodemographic Characteristics of Young Adults Who Value Gluten-Free Food." *Journal of the Academy of Nutrition and Dietetics* 118, no. 8 (August 2018): 1389–1398. doi.org/10.1016/j.jand.2018.04.007.

Carrel, G., L. Egli, C. Tran, P. Schneiter, V. Giusti, D. D'Alessio, and L. Tappy. "Contributions of Fat and Protein to the Incretin Effect of a Mixed Meal." *American Journal of Clinical Nutrition* 94, no. 4 (October 2011): 997–1003. doi:10.3945/ajcn.111.017574.

Clarke, C., and T. Best. "Low-Carbohydrate, High-Fat Dieters: Characteristic Food Choice Motivations, Health Perceptions, and Behaviours." *Food Quality and Preference* 62 (December 2017): 162–171. doi.org/10.1016/j.foodqual.2017.07.006.

Gower, B. A., and A. M. Goss. "The Sliding Set-Point: How Insulin and Diet Interact to Explain the Obesity Epidemic (and How to Fix It)." *Current Opinion in Endocrinology, Diabetes and Obesity* 25, no. 5 (October 2018): 303–309. doi:10.1097/MED.0000000000000426.

Hu, T., L. Yao, K. Reynolds, T. Niu, S. Li, P. Whelton, J. He, and L. Bazzano. "The Effects of a Low-Carbohydrate Diet on Appetite: A Randomized Controlled Trial." *Nutrition, Metabolism, and Cardiovascular Diseases* 26, no. 6 (June 2016): 476–88. doi:10.1016/j.numecd.2015.11.011.

Chapter 4

1. Gropper, S. S., J. L. Smith, and T. P. Carr. *Advanced Nutrition and Human Metabolism*, 7th edition. Boston: Cengage Learning, 2018.

Howell, S., and R. Kones. "'Calories In, Calories Out' and Macronutrient Intake: The Hope, Hype, and Science of Calories." *American Journal of Physiology. Endocrinology and Metabolism* 313, 5 (November 2017): E608–E612. doi:10.1152/ajpendo.00156.2017.

2. Park, M. (2010). "Twinkie Diet Helps Nutrition Professor Lose 27 Pounds." CNN. Accessed November 20, 2018. www.cnn.com/2010/HEALTH/11/08/twinkie.diet.professor/index.html.

3. Gropper et al., 2018.

4. Hall, K. D. "What Is the Required Energy Deficit per Unit Weight Loss?" *International Journal of Obesity* 32, no. 3 (March 2008): 573–576. doi:10.1038/sj.ijo.0803720.

5. Westman, E. C., J. Mavropoulos, W. S. Yancy, and J. S. Volek. "A Review of Low-Carbohydrate Ketogenic Diets." *Current Atherosclerosis Reports* 5, no. 6 (November 2003): 476–483.

6. Miller, T., S. Mull, A. A. Aragon, J. Krieger, and B. J. Schoenfeld. "Resistance Training Combined with Diet Decreases Body Fat while Preserving Lean Mass Independent of Resting Metabolic Rate: A Randomized Trial." *International Journal of Sport Nutrition and Exercise Metabolism* 28, no. 1 (January 2018): 46–54. doi:10.1123/ijsnem.2017-0221.

Jabekk, P. T., I. A. Moe, H. D. Meen, S. E. Tomten, and A. T. Høstmark. "Resistance Training in Overweight Women on a Ketogenic Diet Conserved Lean Body Mass while Reducing Body Fat." *Nutrition and Metabolism* 7, no. 17 (March 2010). doi.org/10.1186/1743-7075-7-17.

7. Sillanpää, E., D. E. Laaksonen, A. Häkkinen, L. Karavirta, B. Jensen, W. J. Kraemer, K. Nyman, et al. "Body Composition, Fitness, and Metabolic Health during Strength and Endurance Training and Their Combination in Middle-Aged and Older Women." *European Journal of Applied Physiology* 106, no. 2 (May 2009): 285–296. doi:10.1007/s00421-009-1013-x.

8. Gropper et al., 2018.

9. Chung, N., M. Y. Park, J. Kim, H. Y. Park, H. Hwang, C. H. Lee, J. S. Han, et al. "Non-Exercise Activity Thermogenesis (NEAT): A Component of Total Daily Energy Expenditure." *Journal of Exercise Nutrition and Biochemistry* 22, no. 2 (June 2018): 23–30. doi:10.20463/jenb.2018.0013.

10. Gropper et al., 2018.

11. Binns, A., M. Gray, and R. Di Brezzo. "Thermic Effect of Food, Exercise, and Total Energy Expenditure in Active Females." *Journal of Science and Medicine in Sport* 18, no. 2 (March 2015): 204–208. doi:10.1016/j.jsams.2014.01.008.

12. Gropper et al., 2018.

13. Antonio, J., D. K. Kalman, J. R. Stout, M. Greenwood, D. S. Willoughby, and G. G. Haff. *Essentials of Sports Nutrition and Supplements.* Totowa, NJ: Humana Press, 2008).

14. Ibid.

15. Van der Louw, E. J., T. J. Williams, B. J. Henry-Barron, J. F. Olieman, J. J. Duvekot, M. J. Vermeulen, N. Bannink, et al. "Ketogenic Diet Therapy for Epilepsy during Pregnancy: A Case Series." *Seizure* 45 (February 2017): 198–201. doi:10.1016/j.seizure.2016.12.019.

16. Gropper et al., 2018.

17. United States Department of Agriculture. "Basic Report: 04053, Oil, Olive, Salad or Cooking." National Nutrient Database for Standard Reference. 2018. Accessed November 26, 2018. Retrieved from ndb.nal.usda.gov.

18. Hall, 2008.

19. Thomas, D. M., C. K. Martin, S. Lettieri, C. Bredlau, K. Kaiser, T. Church, C. Bouchard, et al. "Can a Weight Loss of One Pound a Week Be Achieved with a 3,500-Kcal Deficit? Commentary on a Commonly Accepted Rule." *International Journal of Obesity* 37, no. 12 (December 2013): 1611–1613. doi:10.1038/ijo.2013.51.

20. McDonald, L. *The Women's Book: A Guide to Nutrition, Fat Loss, and Muscle Gain.* Austin, TX: Lyle McDonald Publishing, 2017.

21. Fernández-Elías, V. E., J. F. Ortega, R. K. Nelson, and R. Mora-Rodriguez. "Relationship between Muscle Water and Glycogen Recovery After Prolonged Exercise in the Heat in Humans." *European Journal of Applied Physiology*115, no. 9 (September 2015): 1919–1926. doi:10.1007/s00421-015-3175-z.

22. Ibid.

23. Friedl, K. E., K. A. Westphal, L. J. Marchitelli, J. F. Patton, W. C. Chumlea, and S. Guo. (2001). "Evaluation of Anthropometric Equations to Assess Body-Composition Changes in Young Women." *American Journal of Clinical Nutrition* 73 no. 2 (February 2001): 268–275.

24. Gropper et al. 2018.

Chapter 5

1. Panay, N., and A. Fenton. "The Role of Testosterone in Women." *Climacteric: The Journal of the International Menopause Society* 12, no. 3 (June 2009): 185–187. doi:10.1080/13697130902973227.

2. Liu, T., Y.-Q. Cui, H. Zhao, H.-B. Liu, S.-D. Zhao, Y. Gao, X. L. Mu, et al. "High Levels of Testosterone Inhibit Ovarian Follicle Development By Repressing the FSH Signaling Pathway." *Journal of Huazhong University of Science and Technology* 35, no. 5 (October 2015): 723–729. doi:10.1007/s11596-015-1497-z.

3. Karastergiou, K., S. R. Smith, A. S. Greenberg, and S. K. Fried. "Sex Differences in Human Adipose Tissues—the Biology of Pear Shape." *Biology of Sex Differences* 3, no. 1 (May 2012): 13. doi:10.1186/2042-6410-3-13.

4. Nelson, L. R., and S. E. Bulun. "Estrogen Production and Action." *Journal of the American Academy of Dermatology* 45, no. 3 Supplement (September 2001): S116–S124.

5. Feinshtein, V., Z. Ben-Zvi, E. Sheiner, A. Amash, B. Sheizaf, and G. Holcberg. "Progesterone Levels in Cesarean and Normal Delivered Term Placentas." *Archives of Gynecology and Obstetrics* 281, no. 3 (March 2010): 387–392. doi:10.1007/s00404-009-1125-x.

6. Nelson and Bulun, 2001.

7. Brown, K. A. "Impact of Obesity on Mammary Gland Inflammation and Local Estrogen Production." *Journal of Mammary Gland Biology and Neoplasia* 19, no. 2 (July 2014): 183–189. doi:10.1007/s10911-014-9321-0.

Nelson and Bulun, 2001.

8. American Academy of Pediatrics, American College of Obstetricians and Gynecologists, et al. "Menstruation in Girls and Adolescents: Using the Menstrual Cycle as a Vital Sign." *Pediatrics* 118, no. 5 (November 2006): 2245–2250. doi:10.1542/peds.2006-2481.

Sanfilippo, J. S. "Is the Menstrual Cycle Truly a Vital Sign?" *Journal of Pediatric and Adolescent Gynecology* 27, no. 6 (December 2014): 307–308. doi:10.1016/j.jpag.2014.10.004.

9. Solomon, S. J., M. S. Kurzer, and D. H. Calloway. "Menstrual Cycle and Basal Metabolic Rate in Women." *The American Journal of Clinical Nutrition* 36, no. 4 (October 1982): 611–616. doi:10.1093/ajcn/36.4.611.

10. Ibid.

11. Nagashima, K. "Thermoregulation and Menstrual Cycle." *Temperature* 2, no. 3 (July–September 2015): 320-1. doi:10.1080/23328940.2015.1066926.

12. Kammoun, I., W., Ben Saâda, A. Sifaou, E. Haouat, H. Kandara, L. Ben Salem, and C. Ben Slama. "Change in Women's Eating Habits during the Menstrual Cycle." *Annales d'Endocrinologie* 78, no. 1 (February 2017): 33–37. doi.org/10.1016/j.ando.2016.07.001.

13. Ibid.

14. Gorczyca, A. M., L. A. Sjaarda, E. M. Mitchell, N. J. Perkins, K. C. Schliep, J. Wactawski-Wende, and S. L. Mumford. "Changes in Macronutrient, Micronutrient, and Food Group Intakes throughout the Menstrual Cycle in Healthy, Premenopausal Women." *European Journal of Nutrition* 55, no. 3 (April 2016): 1181–1188. doi:10.1007/s00394-015-0931-0.

15. Gorczyka et al., 2016.

Krishnan, S., K. Agrawal, R. R. Tryon, L. C. Welch, W. F. Horn, J. W. Newman, and N. L. Keim. "Structural Equation Modeling of Food Craving across the Menstrual Cycle Using Behavioral, Neuroendocrine, and Metabolic Factors." *Physiology and Behavior* 195 (October 2018): 28–36. doi:10.1016/j.physbeh.2018.07.011.

16. Barth et al., 2015.

17. Rebello, C. J., and F. L. Greenway. "Reward-Induced Eating: Therapeutic Approaches to Addressing Food Cravings." *Advances in Therapy* 33, no. 11 (November 2016): 1853–1866. doi:10.1007/s12325-016-0414-6.

18. Barth et al., 2015.

19. Escalante and Salazar, 1999.

20. Pereira, R. I., B. A. Casey, T. A. Swibas, C. B. Erickson, P. Wolfe, and R. E. Van Pelt. "Timing of Estradiol Treatment After Menopause May Determine Benefit or Harm to Insulin Action." *Journal of Clinical Endocrinology and Metabolism* 100, no. 12 (December 2015): 4456–4462. doi:10.1210/jc.2015-3084.

21. Escalante and Salazar, 1999.

22. Tai, M. M., T. P. Castillo, and F. X. Pi-Sunyer. "Thermic Effect of Food during Each Phase of the Menstrual Cycle." *American Journal of Clinical Nutrition* 66, no. 5 (November 1997): 1110–1115. doi:10.1093/ajcn/66.5.1110

23. Smith, C. T., Y. Sierra, S. H. Oppler, and C. A. Boettiger. "Ovarian Cycle Effects on Immediate Reward Selection Bias in Humans: A Role for Estradiol." *Journal of Neuroscience* 34, no. 16 (April 2014): 5468–5476. doi:10.1523/JNEUROSCI.0014-14.2014.

24. Krishnan, 2018.

25. White, C. P., C. L. Hitchcock, Y. M. Vigna, and J. C. Prior. "Fluid Retention over the Menstrual Cycle: 1-Year Data from the Prospective Ovulation Cohort." *Obstetrics and Gynecology International* 2011 (2011). dx.doi.org/10.1155/2011/138451.

26. White et al., 2011.

27. Carr-Nangle, R. E., W. G. Johnson, K. C. Bergeron, and D. W. Nangle. "Body Image Changes over the Menstrual Cycle in Normal Women." *International Journal of Eating Disorders* 16, no. 3 (November 1994): 267–273.

Teixeira, A. L. S., M. R. C. Dias, V. O. Damasceno, J. A. Lamounier, and R. M. Gardner. "Association between Different Phases of Menstrual Cycle and Body Image Measures of Perceived Size, Ideal Size, and Body Dissatisfaction." *Perceptual and Motor Skills* 117, no. 3 (December 2013): 892–902. doi:10.2466/24.27.PMS.117x31z1.

28. Teixeira et al., 2013.

29. Ibid.

Patel, S., A. Homaei, A. B. Raju, and B. R. Meher. "Estrogen: The Necessary Evil for Human Health, and Ways to Tame It." *Biomedicine and Pharmacotherapy* 102 (June 2018): 403–411. doi:10.1016/j.biopha.2018.03.078.

30. Ibid.

31. McGrice, M., and J. Porter. "The Effect of Low Carbohydrate Diets on Fertility Hormones and Outcomes in Overweight and Obese Women: A Systematic Review." *Nutrients* 9, no. 3 (February 2017): pii: E204. doi:10.3390/nu9030204.

32. Patel et al., 2018.

33. Ibid.

34. Ibid.

35. Briden, 2017.

36. Patisaul, H. B., and W. Jefferson. "The Pros and Cons of Phytoestrogens." *Frontiers in Neuroendocrinology* 31, no. 4 (October 2010): 400–419. doi:10.1016/j.yfrne.2010.03.003.

Chen, M. N., C. C. Lin, and C. F. Liu. "Efficacy of Phytoestrogens for Menopausal Symptoms: A Meta-Analysis and Systematic Review." *Climacteric: The Journal of the International Menopause Society* 18, no. 2 (April 2015): 260–269. doi:10.3109/13697137.2014.966241.

37. Chen et al., 2015.

38. Handa, Y., H. Fujita, S. Honma, H. Minakami, and R. Kishi. "Estrogen Concentrations in Beef and Human Hormone-Dependent Cancers." *Annals of Oncology* 20, no. 9 (September 2009): 1610–1611 doi.org/10.1093/annonc/mdp381.

39. Ibid.

40. Malekinejad, H., and A. Rezabakhsh. "Hormones in Dairy Foods and Their Impact on Public Health—A Narrative Review Article." *Iranian Journal of Public Health* 44, no. 6 (June 2015): 742–758.

41. Bittner, G. D., M. S. Denison, C. Z. Yang, M. A. Stoner, and G. He. "Chemicals Having Estrogenic Activity Can Be Released from Some Bisphenol A-Free, Hard and Clear, Thermoplastic Resins." *Environmental Health: A Global Access Science Source* 13 (December 2014): 103. doi:10.1186/1476-069X-13-103.

42. National Institute of Environmental Health Sciences. "Bisphenol A (BPA)." National Institute of Environmental Health Sciences. 2018. Accessed December 17, 2018. Retrieved from www.niehs.nih.gov/health/topics/agents/sya-bpa/index.cfm.

43. Mnif, W., A. I. Hassine, A. Bouaziz, A. Bartegi, O. Thomas, and B. Roig. "Effect of Endocrine Disruptor Pesticides: A Review." *International Journal of Environmental Research and Public Health* 8, no. 6 (June 2011): 2265–2303. doi:10.3390/ijerph8062265.

44. Gill, J. "The Effects of Moderate Alcohol Consumption on Female Hormone Levels and Reproductive Function." *Alcohol and Alcoholism* 35, no. 5 (September–October 2000): 417–423 doi.org/10.1093/alcalc/35.5.417.

45. Falsetti, L., E. Pasinetti, M. D. Mazzani, and A. Gastaldi. "Weight Loss and Menstrual Cycle: Clinical and Endocrinological Evaluation." *Gynecological Endocrinology: The Official Journal of the International Society of Gynecological Endocrinology* 6, no. 1 (March 1992): 49–56.

46. Shaw, N. D., S. N. Histed, S. S. Srouji, J. Yang, H. Lee, and J. E. Hall. "Estrogen Negative Feedback on Gonadotropin Secretion: Evidence for a Direct Pituitary Effect in Women." *Journal of Clinical Endocrinology and Metabolism* 95, no. 4 (April 2010): 1955–1961. doi:10.1210/jc.2009-2108.

47. Kumar, P., and S. F. Sait. "Luteinizing Hormone and Its Dilemma in Ovulation Induction." *Journal of Human Reproductive Sciences* 4, no. 1 (January 2011): 2–7. doi:10.4103/0974-1208.82351.

   Mendelson, J. H., N. K. Mello, S. K. Teoh, and J. Ellingboe. "Alcohol Effects on Luteinizing Hormone Releasing Hormone-Stimulated Anterior Pituitary and Gonadal Hormones in Women." *Journal of Pharmacology and Experimental Therapeutics* 250, no. 3 (September 1989): 902–909.

48. Briden, 2017.

49. Wolff, J. "What Doctors Don't Know about Menopause." *AARP.* 2018. Accessed December 17, 2018. Retrieved from www.aarp.org/health/conditions-treatments/info-2018/menopause-symptoms-doctors-relief-treatment.html.

50. Patisaul and Jefferson, 2010.

51. Chen et al., 2014.

52. Grimm, A., A. G. Mensah-Nyagan, and A. Eckert. "Alzheimer, Mitochondria, and Gender." *Neuroscience and Biobehavioral Reviews* 67 (August 2016): 89–101. doi:10.1016/j.neubiorev.2016.04.012.

53. Ibid.

54. La Merrill, M., C. Emond, M. J. Kim, J. P. Antignac, B. Le Bizec, K. Clément, L. S. Birnbaum, et al. "Toxicological Function of Adipose Tissue: Focus on Persistent Organic Pollutants." *Environmental Health Perspectives* 121, no. 2 (February 2013): 162–9. doi:10.1289/ehp.1205485.

55. Ibid.

56. Kim, M. J., P. Marchand, C. Henegar, J. P. Antignac, R. Alili, C. Poitou, et al. "Fate and Complex Pathogenic Effects of Dioxins and Polychlorinated Biphenyls in Obese Subjects before and after Drastic Weight Loss." *Environmental Health Perspectives* 119, no. 3 (March 2011): 377–383. doi:10.1289/ehp.1002848.

57. La Merrill, 2013.

58. McGrice and Porter, 2017.

59. Kulak, D., and A. J. Polotsky. "Should the Ketogenic Diet Be Considered for Enhancing Fertility?" *Maturitas* 74, no. 1 (January 2013): 10–13. doi:10.1016/j.maturitas.2012.10.003.

   Guay, A., and S. R. Davis. "Testosterone Insufficiency in Women: Fact or Fiction?" *World Journal of Urology* 20, no. 2 (June 2002): 106–110. doi:10.1007/s00345-002-0267-2.

   Krishnan, S., R. R. Tryon, W. F. Horn, L. Welch, and N. L. Keim. "Estradiol, SHBG and Leptin Interplay with Food Craving and Intake Across the Menstrual Cycle." *Physiology and Behavior* 165 (October 2016): 304–312. doi:10.1016/j.physbeh.2016.08.010.

Chapter 6

1. Smitka, K., and D. Marešová. "Adipose Tissue as an Endocrine Organ: An Update on Pro-inflammatory and Anti-inflammatory Microenvironment." *Prague Medical Report* 116, no. 2 (2015): 87–111. doi:10.14712/23362936.2015.49.

2. Ibid.

3. Greenwood et al., 2013.

4. Evans P. J., and R. M. Lynch. "Insulin as a Drug of Abuse in Bodybuilding. *British Journal of Sports Medicine* 37, no. 4 (2003): 356–357. dx.doi.org/10.1136/bjsm.37.4.356.

5. Kleiner, 2014.

6. Center for Disease Control, 2017.

7. Ma, X., L. Lin, J. Yue, G. Pradhan, G. Qin, L. J. Minze, H. Wu, et al. "Ghrelin Receptor Regulates HFCS-Induced Adipose Inflammation and Insulin Resistance." *Nutrition and Diabetes* 3 (December 2013): e99. doi:10.1038/nutd.2013.41.

   Teff, K. L., S. S. Elliott, M. Tschöp, T. J. Kieffer, D. Rader, M. Heiman, R. R. Townsend, et al. "Dietary Fructose Reduces Circulating Insulin and Leptin, Attenuates Postprandial Suppression of Ghrelin, and Increases Triglycerides in Women." *Journal of Clinical Endocrinology and Metabolism* 89, no. 6 (June 2004): 2963–2972. doi:10.1210/jc.2003-031855.

8. Lejeune, M. P., K. R., Westerterp, T. C. Adam, N. D. Luscombe-Marsh, and M. S. Westerterp-Plantenga. "Ghrelin and Glucagon-Like Peptide 1 Concentrations, 24-H Satiety, and Energy and Substrate Metabolism during a High-Protein Diet and Measured in a Respiration Chamber." *American Journal of Clinical Nutrition* 83, no. 1 (January 2006): 89–94. doi:10.1093/ajcn/83.1.89.

9. Sumithran, P., L. A. Prendergast, E. Delbridge, K. Purcell, A. Shulkes, A. Kriketos, and J. Proietto. "Ketosis and Appetite-Mediating Nutrients and Hormones after Weight Loss." *European Journal of Clinical Nutrition* 67, no. 7 (July 2013): 759–764. doi:10.1038/ejcn.2013.90.

Paoli, A., G. Bosco, E. M. Camporesi, and D. Mangar. "Ketosis, Ketogenic Diet, and Food Intake Control: A Complex Relationship." *Frontiers in Psychology* 6 (February 2015): 27. doi:10.3389/fpsyg.2015.00027.

10. Sumithran et al., 2013.

11. Volek, J. S., M. J. Sharman, D. M. Love, N. G. Avery, A. L. Gomez, T. P. Scheett, and W. J. Kraemer. "Body Composition and Hormonal Responses to a Carbohydrate-Restricted Diet." *Metabolism: Clinical and Experimental* 51, no. 7 (July 2002): 864–870.

Volek, J. S., S. D. Phinney, C. E. Forsythe, E. E. Quann, R. J. Wood, M. J. Puglisi, W. J. Kraemer, et al. "Carbohydrate Restriction Has a More Favorable Impact on the Metabolic Syndrome than a Low-Fat Diet." *Lipids* 44, no. 4 (April 2009): 297–309. doi:10.1007/s11745-008-3274-2.

Westman, E. C., W. S. Yancy, J. C. Mavropoulos, M. Marquart, and J. R. McDuffie. "The Effect of a Low-Carbohydrate, Ketogenic Diet versus a Low-Glycemic Index Diet on Glycemic Control in Type 2 Diabetes Mellitus." *Nutrition and Metabolism* 5, no. 36 (December 2008). doi:10.1186/1743-7075-5-36.

12. Reynolds, R. C., K. S. Stockmann, F. S. Atkinson, G. S. Denyer, and J. C. Brand-Miller. "Effect of the Glycemic Index of Carbohydrates on Day-Long (10 H) Profiles of Plasma Glucose, Insulin, Cholecystokinin, and Ghrelin." *European Journal of Clinical Nutrition* 63, no. 7 (July 2009): 872–878. doi:10.1038/ejcn.2008.52.

13. Brennan, I. M., K. L. Feltrin, N. S. Nair, T. Hausken, T. J. Little, D. Gentilcore, J. M. Wishart, et al. "Effects of the Phases of the Menstrual Cycle on Gastric Emptying, Glycemia, Plasma GLP-1 and Insulin, and Energy Intake in Healthy Lean Women." *American Journal of Physiology* (Consolidated), 297, no. 3 (September 2009): G602–10. doi:10.1152/ajpgi.00051.2009.

14. Ibid.

15. Kammoun, I., W. Ben Saâda, A. Sifaou, E. Haouat, H. Kandara, L. Ben Salem, and C. Ben Slama. "Change in Women's Eating Habits During the Menstrual Cycle." *Annales d'Endocrinologie* 78, no. 1 (February 2017): 33–37. doi:10.1016/j.ando.2016.07.001.

16. Shiiya, T., M. Nakazato, M. Mizuta, Y. Date, M. S. Mondal, M. Tanaka, S. Nozoe, et al. "Plasma Ghrelin Levels in Lean and Obese Humans and the Effect of Glucose on Ghrelin Secretion." *The Journal of Clinical Endocrinology and Metabolism* 87, no. 1 (January 2002): 240–244. doi:10.1210/jcem.87.1.8129.

17. Gropper, S. S., J. L. Smith, and T. P. Carr. *Advanced Nutrition and Human Metabolism*, 7th edition. Boston: Cengage Learning, 2018.

Iacovides, S., and R. M. Meiring. "The Effect of a Ketogenic Diet versus a High-Carbohydrate, Low-Fat Diet on Sleep, Cognition, Thyroid Function, and Cardiovascular Health Independent of Weight Loss: Study Protocol for a Randomized Controlled Trial." *Trials* 19, no. 1 (January 2018): 62. doi:10.1186/s13063-018-2462-5.

18. Meyer-Gerspach, A. C., B. Wölnerhanssen, B. Beglinger, F. Nessenius, M. Napitupulu, F. H. Schulte, R. E. Stienert et al. "Gastric and Intestinal Satiation in Obese and Normal Weight Healthy People." *Physiology and Behavior* 129 (April 2014): 265–271. doi:10.1016/j.physbeh.2014.02.043.

Geliebter, A. A., and S. A. Hashim. "Gastric Capacity in Normal, Obese, and Bulimic Women." *Physiology and Behavior*, 74, no. 4–5 (November–December 2001): 743–746. doi:10.1016/s0031-9384(01)00619-9.

19. Meyer-Gerspach et al., 2014.

Geliebter and Hashim, 2001.

Latner, J. D., and G. T. Wilson. "Binge Eating and Satiety in Bulimia Nervosa and Binge Eating Disorder: Effects of Macronutrient Intake." *International Journal of Eating Disorders* 36, no. 4 (November 2004): 402–415. doi:10.1002/eat.20060.

20. Geliebter and Hashim, 2001.

21. Latner and Wilson, 2004.

22. Ibid.

23. Lustig, R. H., S. Sen, J. E. Soberman, and P. A. Velasquez-Mieyer. "Obesity, Leptin Resistance, and the Effects of Insulin Reduction." *International Journal of Obesity and Related Metabolic Disorders: Journal of the International Association for the Study of Obesity* 28, no. 10 (October 2001): 1344–1348. doi:10.1038/sj.ijo.0802753.

Martin, S. S., A. Qasim, and M. P. Reilly. "Leptin Resistance: A Possible Interface of Inflammation and Metabolism in Obesity-Related Cardiovascular Disease." *Journal of the American College of Cardiology* 52, no. 15 (October 2008): 1201–1210. doi:10.1016/j.jacc.2008.05.060.

24. Ibid.

25. Baker, J. M., L. Al-Nakkash, and M. M. Herbst-Kralovetz. "Estrogen–Gut Microbiome Axis: Physiological and Clinical Implications." *Maturitas* 103 (September 2017): 45–53. doi:10.1016/j.maturitas.2017.06.025.

Ridlon, J. M., S. Ikegawa, J. M. Alves, B. Zhou, A. Kobayashi, T. Iida, K. Mitamura, et al. "Clostridium Scindens: A Human Gut Microbe with a High Potential to Convert Glucocorticoids into Androgens." *Journal of Lipid Research* 54, no. 9 (September 2013): 2437–2449. doi:10.1194/jlr.M038869.

26. Baker et al., 2017.

27. Ibid.

28. Groh, K. J., B. Geueke, and J. Muncke. "Food Contact Materials and Gut Health: Implications for Toxicity Assessment and Relevance of High Molecular Weight Migrants." *Food and Chemical Toxicology* 109 (Part 1):1–18. doi:10.1016/j.fct.2017.08.023.

29. Wyatt, D. A. "Best Practices vs. Band-Aids for Healing Leaky Gut Syndrome." *Townsend Letter* no. 407 (June 2017): 33.

30. Yan, Y. X., H. B. Xiao, S. S. Wang, J. Zhao, Y. He, W. Wang, and J. Dong. "Investigation of the Relationship between Chronic Stress and Insulin Resistance in a Chinese Population." *Journal of Epidemiology* 26, no. 7 (January 2016): 355–360. doi:10.2188/jea.JE20150183.

31. Ibid.

32. Whitworth, J. A., P. M. Williamson, G. Mangos, and J. J. Kelly. "Cardiovascular Consequences of Cortisol Excess." *Vascular Health and Risk Management* 1, no. 4 (December 2005): 291–299.

33. Ibid.

34. Mohorko, N., M. Černelič-Bizjak, T. Poklar-Vatovec, G. Grom, S. Kenig, A. Petelin, and Z. Jenko-Pražnikar. "Weight Loss, Improved Physical Performance, Cognitive Function, Eating Behavior, and Metabolic Profile in a 12-Week Ketogenic Diet in Obese Adults." *Nutrition Research* 62 (February 2019): 64–77. doi.org/10.1016/j.nutres.2018.11.007.

35. Ibid.

36. Mullur, R., Y. Y. Liu, and G. A. Brent. "Thyroid Hormone Regulation of Metabolism." *Physiological Reviews* 94, no. 2 (April 2014): 355–382. doi:10.1152/physrev.00030.2013.

37. Ibid.

38. Ibid.

39. Tahboub, R., and B. M. Arafah. "Sex Steroids and the Thyroid." *Best Practice and Research: Clinical Endocrinology and Metabolism* 23, no. 6 (December 2009): 769–780. doi:10.1016/j.beem.2009.06.005.

40. Patel, S., A. Homaei, A. B. Raju, and B. R. Meher. "Estrogen: The Necessary Evil for Human Health, and Ways to Tame It." *Biomedicine and Pharmacotherapy* 102 (June 2018): 403–411. doi:10.1016/j.biopha.2018.03.078.

41. Mathieson, R. A., J. L. Walberg, F. C. Gwazdauskas, D. E. Hinkle, and J. M. Gregg. "The Effect of Varying Carbohydrate Content of a Very-Low-Caloric Diet on Resting Metabolic Rate and Thyroid Hormones." *Metabolism: Clinical and Experimental* 35, no. 5 (May 1986): 394–398.

42. Phinney, S. "Does Your Thyroid Need Dietary Carbohydrates?" *Virta*. May 3, 2017. Accessed Dec. 29, 2018. Retrieved from blog.virtahealth.com/does-your-thyroid-need-dietary-carbohydrates.

43. Ibid.

44. Shanahan, C. "Going Low-Carb Too Fast May Trigger Thyroid Troubles and Hormone Imbalance." *Dr. Cate*. February 26, 2012. Accessed December 28, 2018. Retrieved from drcate.com/going-low-carb-too-fast-may-trigger-thyroid-troubles-and-hormone-imbalance.

Luis, D., J. C. Domingo, O. Izaola, F. F. Casanueva, D. Bellido, and I. Sajoux. "Effect of DHA Supplementation in a Very Low-Calorie Ketogenic Diet in the Treatment of Obesity: A Randomized Clinical Trial." *Endocrine* 54, no. 1 (October 2016): 111–122. doi:10.1007/s12020-016-0964-z.

Meier, U., and A. M. Gressner. "Endocrine Regulation of Energy Metabolism: Review of Pathobiochemical and Clinical Chemical Aspects of Leptin, Ghrelin, Adiponectin, and Resistin." *Clinical Chemistry* 50, no. 9 (September 2004):1511–25. doi:10.1373/clinchem.2004.032482.

Centers for Disease Control and Prevention. "National Diabetes Statistics Report." Centers for Disease Control and Prevention, 2017. Accessed October 30, 2018. Retrieved from www.cdc.gov/diabetes/data/statistics/statistics-report.html.

Sapolsky, R. *Why Zebras Don't Get Ulcers: The Acclaimed Guide to Stress, Stress-Related Diseases, and Coping*, 3rd edition. New York: Holt Paperbacks, 2004.

Chapter 7

1. Sillanpää, E., D. E. Laaksonen, A. Häkkinen, L. Karavirta, B. Jensen, W. J. Kraemer, K. Nyman, et al. "Body Composition, Fitness, and Metabolic Health during Strength and Endurance Training and Their Combination in Middle-Aged and Older Women." *European Journal of Applied Physiology* 106, no. 2 (May 2009): 285–296. doi:10.1007/s00421-009-1013-x.

2. Miller, T., S. Mull, A. A. Aragon, J. Krieger, and B. J. Schoenfeld. "Resistance Training Combined with Diet Decreases Body Fat while Preserving Lean Mass Independent of Resting Metabolic Rate: A Randomized Trial." *International Journal of Sport Nutrition and Exercise Metabolism* 28, no. 1 (January 2018): 46–54. doi:10.1123/ijsnem.2017-0221.

Jabekk, P. T., I. A. Moe, H. D. Meen, S. E. Tomten, and A. T. Høstmark. "Resistance Training in Overweight Women on a Ketogenic Diet Conserved Lean Body Mass while Reducing Body Fat." *Nutrition and Metabolism* 7, no. 17 (March 2010). doi.org/10.1186/1743-7075-7-17.

3. Stavres, J., M. Zeigler, and M. Bayles. "Six Weeks of Moderate Functional Resistance Training Increases Basal Metabolic Rate in Sedentary Adult Women." *International Journal of Exercise Science* 11, no. 2 (January 2018): 32–41.

4. McGarrah, R. W., C. A. Slentz, and W. E. Kraus. "The Effect of Vigorous-versus Moderate-Intensity Aerobic Exercise on Insulin Action." *Current Cardiology Reports* 18, no. 12 (December 2016): 117. doi:10.1007/s11886-016-0797-7.

5. Ibid.

6. Clow, A., and S. Edmunds. *Physical Activity and Mental Health.* Champaign, IL: Human Kinetics, Inc., 2014.

7. Copeland, J. L., L. A. Consitt, and M. S Tremblay. "Hormonal Responses to Endurance and Resistance Exercise in Females Aged 19–69 Years." *The Journals of Gerontology Series A,* 57, no. 4 (April 2002): B158–B165.

8. Ibid.

9. Volek, J., E. Quann, and C. Forsythe. "Low-Carbohydrate Diets Promote a More Favorable Body Composition than Low-Fat Diets." *Strength and Conditioning Journal* 32, no. 1 (February 2010): 42–47. doi:10.1519/SSC.0b013e3181c16c41.

10. Ibid.

11. Ibid.

12. Volek, J. S., and S. D. Phinney. *The Art and Science of Low Carbohydrate Performance.* Miami: Beyond Obesity LLC, 2012.

13. Wroble, K. A., M. N. Trott, G. G. Schweitzer, R. S. Rahman, P. V. Kelly, and E. P. Weiss. "Low-Carbohydrate, Ketogenic Diet Impairs Anaerobic Exercise Performance in Exercise-Trained Women and Men: A Randomized-Sequence Crossover Trial." *Journal of Sports Medicine and Physical Fitness* (April 2018). doi:10.23736/S0022-4707.18.08318-4.

14. Volek and Phinney, 2012.

15. D'eon, T., and B. Braun. "The Roles of Estrogen and Progesterone in Regulating Carbohydrate and Fat Utilization at Rest and during Exercise." *Journal of Women's Health and Gender-Based Medicine* 11, no. 3 (April 2002): 225–237. doi:10.1089/152460902753668439.

16. Peric, R., M. Meucci, and Z. Nikolovski. "Fat Utilization during High-Intensity Exercise: When Does It End?" *Sports Medicine—Open* 2, no. 1 (December 2016): 35. doi:10.1186/s40798-016-0060-1.

17. Ibid.

18. Cox, P. J., T. Kirk, T. Ashmore, K. Willerton, R. Evans, A. Smith, A. J. Murray, et al. "Nutritional Ketosis Alters Fuel Preference and Thereby Endurance Performance in Athletes." *Cell Metabolism* 24, no. 2 (August 2016): 256–268. doi:10.1016/j.cmet.2016.07.010.

19. Greene, D. A., B. J. Varley, T. B. Hartwig, P. Chapman, and M. Rigney. "A Low-Carbohydrate Ketogenic Diet Reduces Body Mass without Compromising Performance in Powerlifting and Olympic Weightlifting Athletes." *Journal of Strength and Conditioning Research* 32, no. 12 (December 2018): 3373–3382. doi:10.1519/JSC.0000000000002904.

20. Ibid.

21. Ibid.

22. Salvatore, J., and J. Marecek. "Gender in the Gym: Evaluation Concerns as Barriers to Women's Weight Lifting." *Sex Roles* 63, no. 7–8 (October 2010): 556–557. doi.org/10.1007/s11199-010-9800-8.

23. Volek et al., 2010.

24. Salvatore and Marecek, 2010.

25. Ibid.

26. Ibid.

27. Jabekk, 2010; Stavres et al., 2018.

28. Migala, J. "Halle Berry Swears By The Keto Diet—Here's Exactly What She Eats." *Women's Health.* 2018. Accessed 01/07/2019. Retrieved from www.womenshealthmag.com/weight-loss/a22000172/halle-berry-keto-diet.

29. Antonio, J., D. K. Kalman, J. R. Stout, M. Greenwood, D. S. Willoughby, and G. G. Haff. *Essentials of Sports Nutrition and Supplements.* Totowa, NJ: Humana Press, 2008.

30. Ibid.

Chapter 8

1. Trepanowski, J. F., and K. A. Varady. "A Diet with Carbohydrates Eaten Primarily at Dinner: An Innovative, Nutritional Approach to End the Vicious Cycle of Abdominal Obesity." In Watson, R. E., ed., *Nutrition in the Prevention and Treatment of Abdominal Obesity.* Cambridge, MA: Academic Press, 2014. 401–414.

2. Nishino, K., M. Sakurai, Y. Takeshita, and T. Takamura. "Consuming Carbohydrates after Meat or Vegetables Lowers Postprandial Excursions of Glucose and Insulin in Nondiabetic Subjects." *Journal of Nutritional Science and Vitaminology* 64, no. 5 (2018): 316–320. doi:10.3177/jnsv.64.316.

3. Fernández-Elías, V. E., J. F. Ortega, R. K. Nelson, and R. Mora-Rodriguez. "Relationship between Muscle Water and Glycogen Recovery after Prolonged Exercise in the Heat in Humans." *European Journal of Applied Physiology* 115, no. 9 (September 2015): 1919–1926. doi:10.1007/s00421-015-3175-z.

4. Seimon, R. V., J. A. Roekenes, J. Zibellini, B. Zhu, A. A, Gibson, A. P, Hills, R. E. Wood, et al. "Do Intermittent Diets Provide Physiological Benefits over Continuous Diets for Weight Loss? A Systematic Review of Clinical Trials." *Molecular and Cellular Endocrinology,* 418 Part 2 (December 2015) 153–172. doi:10.1016/j.mce.2015.09.014.

5. Miller, T., S. Mull, A. A. Aragon, J. Krieger, and B. J. Schoenfeld. "Resistance Training Combined with Diet Decreases Body Fat while Preserving Lean Mass Independent of Resting Metabolic Rate: A Randomized Trial." *International Journal of Sport Nutrition and Exercise Metabolism* 28, no. 1 (January 2018): 46–54. doi:10.1123/ijsnem.2017-0221.

Chapter 9

1. Namazi, N., S. Aliasgharzadeh, R. Mahdavi, and F. Kolahdooz. "Accuracy of the Common Predictive Equations for Estimating Resting Energy Expenditure among Normal and Overweight Girl University Students." *Journal of the American College of Nutrition* 35, no. 2 (2016) 136–142. doi:10.1080/07315724.2014.938280.

2. Gropper, S., J. Smith, and T. Carr. *Advanced Nutrition and Human Metabolism*, 7th edition. Boston: Cengage Learning, 2018.

3. Ibid.

4. Seimon, R. V., J. A. Roekenes, J. Zibellini, B. Zhu, A. A, Gibson, A. P, Hills, R. E. Wood, et al. "Do Intermittent Diets Provide Physiological Benefits over Continuous Diets for Weight Loss? A Systematic Review of Clinical Trials." *Molecular and Cellular Endocrinology*, 418 Part 2 (December 2015) 153–172. doi:10.1016/j.mce.2015.09.014.

5. Trepanowski, J. F., and K. A. Varady. "Intermittent Versus Daily Calorie Restriction in Visceral Fat Loss." In Watson, R. E., ed., *Nutrition in the Prevention and Treatment of Abdominal Obesity*. Cambridge, MA: Academic Press, 2014. 181–188.

6. Institute of Medicine. *Dietary Reference Intakes for Energy, Carbohydrate, Fiber, Fat, Fatty Acids, Cholesterol, Protein, and Amino Acids*. Washington, DC: The National Academies Press, 2005.

7. Volek, J. S., and S. D. Phinney. *The Art and Science of Low Carbohydrate Performance*. Miami: Beyond Obesity LLC, 2012.

8. Friedl, K. E., K. A. Westphal, L. J. Marchitelli, J. F. Patton, W. C. Chumlea, and S. Guo. (2001). "Evaluation of Anthropometric Equations to Assess Body-Composition Changes in Young Women." *American Journal of Clinical Nutrition*, 73, no. 2 (February 2001): 268–275.

9. Ljubicic, M., M. M. Saric, I. Rumbak, I. C. Baric, D. Komes, Z. Satalic, and R. P. F. Guiné. "Knowledge about Dietary Fibre and Its Health Benefits: A Cross-Sectional Survey of 2,536 Residents from across Croatia." *Medical Hypotheses* 105 (August 2017): 25–31. doi:10.1016/j.mehy.2017.06.019.

Chapter 10

1. Volek, J. S., S. D Phinney. *The Art and Science of Low Carbohydrate Performance*. Miami: Beyond Obesity LLC, 2012.

   Westman, E. C., J. Mavropoulos, W. S. Yancy, and J. S. Volek. "A Review of Low-Carbohydrate Ketogenic Diets." *Current Atherosclerosis Reports* 5, no. 6 (November 2003): 476–483.

Chapter 11

1. Simopoulos, A. "The Importance of the Ratio of Omega-6/Omega-3 Essential Fatty Acids." *Biomedicine and Pharmacotherapy* 56, no. 8 (October 2002): 365–379.

2. Lands, B., D. Bibus, and K. D. Stark. "Dynamic Interactions of n-3 and n-6 Fatty Acid Nutrients." *Prostaglandins, Leukotrienes and Essential Fatty Acids (PLEFA)* 136 (September 2018): 15–21. doi:10.1016/j.plefa.2017.01.012.

3. Ibid.

4. Hardman, E. "Omega-3 Fatty Acids to Augment Cancer Therapy." *Journal of Nutrition* 132, no. 11 Supplement (November 2002): 3508S–3512S. doi:10.1093/jn/132.11.3508S.

5. Freeman, M. P., J. R. Hibbeln, M. Silver, A. M. Hirschberg, B. Wang, A. M. Yule, L. F. Petrillo, et al. "Omega-3 Fatty Acids for Major Depressive Disorder Associated with the Menopausal Transition: A Preliminary Open Trial." *Menopause* 18, no. 3 March 2011): 279–284. doi:10.1097/gme.0b013e3181f2ea2e.

6. Ibid.

7. Zafari, M., F. Behmanesh, and A. Agha Mohammadi. (2011). "Comparison of the Effect of Fish Oil and Ibuprofen on Treatment of Severe Pain in Primary Dysmenorrhea." *Caspian Journal of Internal Medicine* 2, no. 3 (Summer 2011): 279–282.

8. Orchard, T. S., X. Pan, F. Cheek, S. W. Ing, and R. D. Jackson. "A Systematic Review of Omega-3 Fatty Acids and Osteoporosis." *British Journal of Nutrition* 107 Supplement 2, no. 2 (June 2012): S253–S260. doi:10.1017/S0007114512001638.

9. Nadjarzadeh, A., R. Dehghani Firouzabadi, N. Vaziri, H. Daneshbodi, M. H. Lotfi, and H. Mozaffari-Khosravi. "The Effect of Omega-3 Supplementation on Androgen Profile and Menstrual Status in Women with Polycystic Ovary Syndrome: A Randomized Clinical Trial." *Iranian Journal of Reproductive Medicine* 11, no. 8 (August 2013): 665–672.

10. Ibid.

11. Donnelly, J. K., and D. S. Robinson. "Free Radicals in Foods." *Free Radical Research* 22, no. 2 (February 1995): 147–176.

12. Sanfilippo, D. *Practical Paleo*. Las Vegas, NV: Victory Belt Publishing, 2016.

13. U.S. Food and Drug Administration. "Final Determination Regarding Partially Hydrogenated Oils (Removing Trans Fat)." U.S. Food and Drug Administration. 2018. Accessed November 1, 2018. Retrieved from www.fda.gov/food/ ingredientspackaginglabeling /foodadditivesingredients /ucm449162.htm.

14. World Health Organization. News Release: "WHO Plan to Eliminate Industrially Produced Trans-Fatty Acids from Global Food Supply. World Health Organization, May 2018. Retrieved from www.who.int /news-room/detail/14-05-2018- who-plan-to-eliminate-industrially- produced-trans-fatty-acids-from- global-food-supply.

15. Malekinejad, H., and A. Rezabakhsh. "Hormones in Dairy Foods and Their Impact on Public Health—A Narrative Review Article." *Iranian Journal of Public Health* 44, no. 6 (June 2015): 742–758.

16. U.S. Food and Drug Administration. "Final Determination Regarding Partially Hydrogenated Oils (Removing Trans Fat)." U.S. Food and Drug Administration, 2018. Accessed Nov. 1, 2018. Retrieved from www.fda.gov/food/ ingredientspackaginglabeling /foodadditivesingredients /ucm449162.htm.

17. Metcalf, T. "Keto Taco Seasoning Recipe." Ketogasm. 2018. Retrieved from ketogasm.com/ keto-taco-seasoning-recipe.

18. Ter Horst, K. W., and M. J. Serlie. "Fructose Consumption, Lipogenesis, and Non-Alcoholic Fatty Liver Disease." *Nutrients* 9, no. 9 (September 2017): ii. E981. doi:10.3390/nu9090981.

19. UW Health. "Fructose-Restricted Diet." University of Wisconsin Hospital and Clinics Authority. 2015. Retrieved from www.uwhealth.org/ healthfacts/nutrition/376.pdf.

20. McDonald, L. *The Ketogenic Diet: A Complete Guide for the Dieter and Practitioner.* Austin, TX: Lyle McDonald Publishing, 1998.

21. Zakhari, S. (2006). "Overview: How Is Alcohol Metabolized by the Body?" *Alcohol Research and Health: The Journal of the National Institute of Alcohol Abuse and Alcoholism* 29, no. 4 (February 2006): 245–254.

22. Ibid.

23. Baumer, E. M. "Using the Zimbabwe Hand Teaching Method with an Urban Austrian Population." *Diabetes Spectrum* 12, no. 3 (1999): 185.

24. Ibid.

25. Ibid.

    National Nutrient Database for Standard Reference Legacy Release. "Basic Report: 09030, Apricots, Dehydrated (Low-Moisture), Sulfured, Uncooked. United States Department of Agriculture. 2018.

    National Nutrient Database for Standard Reference Legacy Release. "Basic Report: 09021, Apricots, Raw." United States Department of Agriculture. 2018.

Chapter 12

1. Pooralajal et al., 2017.

2. Horita, S., G. Seki, H. Yamada, M. Suzuki, K. Koike, and T. Fujita. "Insulin Resistance, Obesity, Hypertension, and Renal Sodium Transport." *International Journal of Hypertension* 2011 (2011):391762. doi:10.4061/2011/391762.

3. Sigler M. H. "The Mechanism of the Natriuresis of Fasting." *Journal of Clinical Investigation* 55, no. 2 (February 1975): 377–387.

4. Institute of Medicine. *Dietary Reference Intakes for Water, Potassium, Sodium, Chloride, and Sulfate.* Washington, DC: The National Academies Press, 2005.

5. Ibid.

6. Institute of Medicine, 2005.

7. National Institutes of Health, 2018.

8. Ibid.

9. Cuciureanu, M.D., and R. Vink. "Magnesium and Stress." From Vink, R. and M. Nechifor, eds, *Magnesium in the Central Nervous System.* Adelaide, Australia: University of Adelaide Press, 2011.

10. Woolhouse, M. "Migraine and Tension Headache—A Complementary and Alternative Medicine Approach." *Australian Family Physician* 34, no. 8 (August 2005): 647–651.

11. National Institutes of Health, 2016.

12. Uysal, N., S. Kizildag, Z. Yuce, G. Guvendi, S. Kandis, B. Koc, A. Karakilic, et al. "Timeline (Bioavailability) of Magnesium Compounds in Hours: Which Magnesium Compound Works Best?" *Biological Trace Element Research* 187, no. 1 (January 2019): 128–136. doi:10.1007 /s12011-018-1351-9.

13. National Institutes of Health, 2016.

14. Ibid.

15. Ibid.

16. Ibid.

17. Ibid.

18. Ibid.

19. Ibid.

20. Romagnoli, E., M. Mascia, C. Cipriani, V. Fassino, F. Mazzei, E. D'Erasmo, V., Carnevale, et al. "Short and Long-Term Variations in Serum Calciotropic Hormones after a Single Very Large Dose of Ergocalciferol (Vitamin D2) or Cholecalciferol (Vitamin D3) in the Elderly." *Journal of Clinical Endocrinology and Metabolism* 93, no. 8 (August 2008): 3015–3020. doi:10.1210/jc.2008-0350.

21. Institute of Medicine. *Dietary Reference Intakes for Calcium, Phosphorus, Magnesium, Vitamin D, and Fluoride.* Washington, DC: The National Academies Press, 1997.

22. National Institutes of Health, 2016.

23. American Thyroid Association. "American Thyroid Association (ATA) Issues Statement on the Potential Risks of Excess Iodine Ingestion and Exposure." American Thyroid Association. 2013. Retrieved from www.thyroid.org/american-thyroid-association-ata-issues-statement-on-the-potential-risks-of-excess-iodine-ingestion-and-exposure.

Ventura, M., M. Melo, and F. Carrilho. "Selenium and Thyroid Disease: From Pathophysiology to Treatment." *International Journal of Endocrinology* 2017 (2017). doi:10.1155/2017/1297658.

24. National Institutes of Health, 2016.

25. American Thyroid Association, 2013.

26. Ventura et al., 2017.

National Institutes of Health Office of Dietary Supplements. "Calcium: Fact Sheet for Consumers." Bethesda, MD: U.S. Department of Health and Human Services, 2016. Retrieved from ods.od.nih.gov/factsheets/Calcium-Consumer.

National Institutes of Health Office of Dietary Supplements. "Iodine: Fact Sheet for Consumers." Bethesda, MD: U.S. Department of Health and Human Services, 2016. Retrieved from ods.od.nih.gov/factsheets/Iodine-Consumer.

National Institutes of Health Office of Dietary Supplements. "Iron: Fact Sheet for Consumers." Bethesda, MD: U.S. Department of Health and Human Services, 2016. Retrieved from ods.od.nih.gov/factsheets/Iron-Consumer.

National Institutes of Health Office of Dietary Supplements. "Magnesium: Fact Sheet for Consumers." Bethesda, MD: U.S. Department of Health and Human Services, 2016. Retrieved from ods.od.nih.gov/factsheets/Magnesium-Consumer.

National Institutes of Health Office of Dietary Supplements. "Potassium: Fact Sheet for Consumers." Bethesda, MD: U.S. Department of Health and Human Services, 2018. Retrieved from ods.od.nih.gov/factsheets/Potassium-Consumer.

National Institutes of Health Office of Dietary Supplements. "Vitamin D: Fact Sheet for Consumers." Bethesda, MD: U.S. Department of Health and Human Services, 2016. Retrieved from ods.od.nih.gov/factsheets/VitaminD-Consumer

Wyatt, D. A. "Best Practices vs. Band-Aids for Healing Leaky Gut Syndrome." *Townsend Letter* no. 407 (June 2017): 33.

About the Author

Tasha Metcalf is a nutrition writer and educator who specializes in helping women ditch the one-size-fits–all diet mind-set to develop a personalized approach to keto and create sustainable, healthy eating habits. She is the owner and founder of Ketogasm, a wildly popular website and resource for women learning to implement a ketogenic diet. Tasha has an extensive science background, having earned a biology degree and studied nutrition at the graduate level.

Tasha has followed a ketogenic diet intermittently since 2011 to heal hormonal imbalances, overcome health issues, and maintain a healthy weight. She shares her meals, recipes, and tips on her site and social media, where she keeps things lighthearted and fun. Tasha also teaches the well-known Hello Keto course and online nutrition workshops.

She lives in Tacoma, Washington, with her partner, Bradley, and their two amazing kiddos.

Gratitude

Writing a book is more challenging than I had anticipated but more fulfilling than I could have possibly imagined. I have to take a moment to thank all the people who helped make this book possible. Without you, it would be stuck rattling around inside my head—a "what if," a "one day," an unchecked box on my bucket list. From the bottom of my heart, thank you all for helping make my vision a reality.

I start by thanking my publisher and the hardworking team at Quarto for bringing this book together. There is so much behind-the-scenes work that goes into making a book—editing, designing, marketing, production, logistics, sales—writing the darned thing was just one small piece of the puzzle. Special thanks to Jill Alexander for championing this project from the start and providing insightful feedback along the way. Tiffany Hill, Anne Re, Todd Conly, and everyone involved in getting this book out there—thank you all for your help with this process. I am truly honored to be a part of the Quarto family. Let's make more books!

To my children, Sebina and Felix, for bringing me joy beyond my wildest dreams. For keeping a smile on my face and giving me a reason to push forward during trying times. For being my "why" in every pursuit. I love you both more than you will ever know.

I am eternally grateful for my mom and dad, Lisa and Steve, for loving me fiercely and always encouraging me to pursue my passions. Thank you for your unwavering support in all of my endeavors—big and small. For raising me to take chances and believe that "you never know unless you try." And, of course, thank you for putting me on this Earth . . . I literally wouldn't be here without you!

To my partner, Bradley, thank you for always being there for our family. Ups, downs, ins, outs, you are our rock and such a wonderful daddy. For encouraging me to step outside my comfort zone, entertaining my crazy ideas, telling the best jokes, and laughing at my bad ones. Thank you for helping me juggle all things by taking on more to help me stay on track and maintain my sanity. You are seriously the best!

To my sister, Tiffany, thank you for everything! For being my twin with three candy necklaces and keeping years of inside jokes alive. For cheering me on when I needed it the most. For reading each chapter, giving honest feedback, and instilling in me a genuine appreciation for the Oxford comma. Thank you for keeping the site and social media thriving while I retreated into my office for months on end.

Huge thanks to my brother, Trevor, for being an absolute genius and sharing your tech savvy with me. Thank you for taking time to develop the supplemental calculator for the book and sparing me from learning any more coding than I need to! Best. Keto calculator. Ever!

To my second mama, Viola, thank you for seeing past my façade to offer help when I was too stubborn to ask for it. For helping me bring order to an endlessly chaotic house and for being the Gram that makes every day an adventure. Thank you for giving me reminders to take breaks and celebrate my accomplishments.

To my LNH crew—I love you all and miss you more than ever.

To the teachers at Children of Hope, it really does take a village! A tremendous thank you to Tifhany Jones, Ella Jackson, Heidi Gibson, Sandy Franks, and Shaneika McDonald for providing such a loving, positive learning environment for my little ones. We are truly blessed to be a part of your warm, caring community. Words do not begin to express my gratitude and appreciation for all you have done for my children and our family as I transitioned careers, returned to grad school, and pursued my dreams. You are all amazing!

And last, but certainly not least, thank you to the most badass keto babes I have ever had the pleasure of meeting. Thank you for building a supportive keto community for women with me, for sharing your knowledge and experience, for creating learning resources, and for gracefully tolerating internet trolls. Casie Ann Cameron, Dori Cameron Ortman, Julia Sweet, Katrina Sager, Kelle Thomsen, Maria Garzon, Tammy Carver, and Teddy Curle—y'all are the real MVPs! I am so grateful for your time and help, but, most importantly, your friendships. Thanks a million, you guys!

General Index

Recipe Index